Oral Medical English in Clinical Practice

临床医学英语口语

主编 ◎ 黄 刚 徐俊波

西南交通大学出版社

·成都·

图书在版编目（CIP）数据

临床医学英语口语 / 黄刚，徐俊波主编. —成都：
西南交通大学出版社，2021.8
ISBN 978-7-5643-8197-4

Ⅰ. ①临… Ⅱ. ①黄… ②徐… Ⅲ. ①临床医学 – 英
语 – 口语 – 医学院校 – 教材 Ⅳ. ①R4

中国版本图书馆 CIP 数据核字（2021）第 164760 号

Linchuang Yixue Yingyu Kouyu
临床医学英语口语

主编 黄　刚　徐俊波

责任编辑　牛　君
封面设计　原谋书装
出版发行　西南交通大学出版社
　　　　　（四川省成都市二环路北一段 111 号
　　　　　西南交通大学创新大厦 21 楼）
发行部电话　028-87600564　87600533
邮政编码　610031
网址　http://www.xnjdcbs.com
印刷　四川煤田地质制图印刷厂
成品尺寸　146 mm × 208 mm
印张　8.25
字数　298 千
版次　2021 年 8 月第 1 版
印次　2021 年 8 月第 1 次
书号　ISBN 978-7-5643-8197-4
定价　28.00 元

课件咨询电话：028-81435775
图书如有印装质量问题　本社负责退换
版权所有　盗版必究　举报电话：028-87600562

编　委　会

F 序
oreword

　　在日新月异的循征医学时代，如何及时高效地获得最新、可靠的专业知识是广大临床医师保持、提升自己专业水平的重要挑战。作为一门工具性的学科，医学专业英语对临床医师阅读英语文献、了解国外最新进展、更好地与国外同行进行学术交流具有重要作用。笔者 1988—1991 年在美国波士顿大学做高访学者，在 Framingham 心脏研究所担任研究员期间，及数十年与国外同道的学术交流中，深感医学英语对现代医师，在医患沟通与学术交流中不可或缺，其重要性不亚于专业知识本身。但近年来寻访书肆，却难觅实用性强的医学专业英语书籍以供参考，专业英语的学习之路倍加困难，尤以口语表达最为突出。当今国内同道已能在国际一流期刊发表具有相当学术影响力的论文，但普遍的弱点仍在于口语，心中纵有万千语，却难以道出。

近日喜见俊波教授和黄刚博士主编的《临床医学英语口语》，令人耳目一新。与其他医学英语书籍最大的不同处在于：该书结合医患沟通、医疗交流等日常临床工作场景，从词汇、句型、对话等方面介绍了医学英语的应用，临床实用性突出，可视为一本简略版"医学英语口语指南"，读者在熟知各临床工作场景中的典型句型和例句基础上加以揣摩练习，假以时日便可灵活应用于日常涉外临床工作中。

两位主编曾分别在德奥两国长期学习、工作，李惠君医生亦在美国半岛医学中心执业行医，他们对欧美多文化、多语言的临床工作环境有着宝贵的直接心得体会，相信该书必能为广大读者提升临床医学英语实践能力助一臂之力。

中国高血压特殊贡献奖得主
第二届"中国医师奖"获得者
张廷杰
2021 年 5 月于成都

　　医学英语可以说是一门全新的语言，因其大量专业词汇来源于拉丁语和希腊语，对以英语为母语的欧美医学生尚有一定难度，更不用说非英语母语的医学生。语言的功能属性是交流，学习任何一门外语也应"学以致用"。母语的自然学习过程是由听说到读写，而多数国人学习外语是从读写到听说，因而不可避免地存在听说能力相对弱于读写能力的尴尬。在现代医学时代，掌握医学专业英语不仅有利于医学生、医务工作者专业知识的更新，也有利于开展临床涉外医疗，更有利于对外医学学术交流协助拓展深入。临床医学是一门以患者为中心的实践科学，日常工作中涉及医患、医护以及其他人员的各种交流沟通。西医先驱 William Osler 就曾说道："Just listen to your patient, he is telling you the diagnosis."而良好的医学英语表达沟通能力也是一名优秀临床医师所必备的基本职业素养。

　　本书内容贴近临床实践，侧重临床医学英语听说，突出临床实践中的口语表达难点和"实用"的特点。与传统医学英语书籍重点关注理论相比，本书以"词汇—句子—对话"的方式介绍日常临床医学英语，配有大量例句和情景对话，以在示范的基础上达到"举一反三、触类旁通"的效果，同时读者通过模仿训练可逐步形成自己的交流方式。本书适用于各级临床医师、临床医学研究生和本科生，使用过程中尤其应注意基础词汇、关键动词及常用句型的用法。本书对重要的专业词汇配有汉语翻译，但需注意潜意识汉语思维的影响。

本书重点关注临床医疗工作中口语交流所需，并未涵盖医学英语的其他内容，也未涉及临床医学亚专业的医学英语，挂一漏万，在所难免，欢迎专家与读者不吝赐教，以利再版时补充和更正。

本书编写过程中得到了西南交通大学医学院及成都市第三人民医院（西南交通大学附属医院）同仁们的热情关心和帮助，研究生游月婷、张悦及刘晓翰参与了部分编务工作，在此谨表谢忱。

编者

2021 年 5 月

C目录
ontents

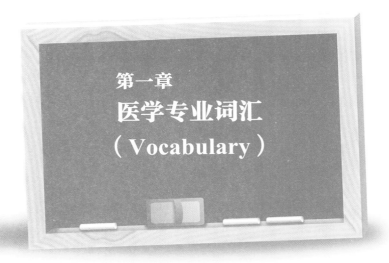

第一章
医学专业词汇
（Vocabulary）

Wherever the art of Medicine is loved,

there is also a love of Humanity.

— Hippocrates

医学专业词汇多源于拉丁语及希腊语，其构词的典型方式为前缀+连接元音(多为 O)+词根+连接元音(O)+后缀。前后缀及词根在专业词汇的构成中具有重要作用，掌握好以它们为基础的专业词汇构词法及一定数量的各医学亚专业词汇，有利于医学专业英语的学习和应用。

第一节　词根（Roots）

一个医学专业单词中，可以有一个或者多个词根，它们通过元音与前缀、后缀连接，构成一个完整单词。

一、器官/部位词根（Roots for Organs & Body Parts）

Abdomen (腹部):
abdomin/o (abdominal 腹部的), lapar/o (laparoscopy 腹腔镜检查), celi/o (celiac 腹腔的)

Backbone (脊柱):
vertebr/o (vertebral 脊椎的), spondyl/o (spondylitis 脊柱炎), spin/o (spinal column 脊柱)

Urinary bladder (膀胱):
vesic/o (vesical 膀胱的), cyst/o (cystitis 膀胱炎)

Blood vessel (血管):
angi/o (angiogram 血管造影), vas/o (vasoconstriction 血管收缩), vascul/o (vascular 血管的)

Breast (乳房):
mamm/o (mammogram 乳房钼靶片), mast/o (mastectomy 乳房切除术)

Eardrum (鼓膜):
tympan/o (tympanic 鼓膜的), myring/o (myringotomy 鼓膜切开术)

Eye (眼):

ocul/o (ocular 视觉的), ophthalm/o (ophthalmoscope 检眼镜), opt/o (optician 验光师), optic/o (optical 视觉的)

Heart (心):

coron/o (coronary 冠状动脉), cardi/o (cardiology 心脏病学)

Kidney (肾):

ren/o (renal 肾脏的), nephr/o (nephritis 肾炎)

Lung (肺):

pulmon/o (pulmonary 肺的), pneumon/o (pneumonectomy 肺切除术), pulm/o (pulmoaortic 肺主动脉的)

Mouth (口):

or/o (oral 口腔的), stomat/o (stomatitis 口腔炎)

Muscle (肌肉):

muscul/o (muscular 肌肉的), my/o (myoma 肌瘤), myos/o (myositis 肌炎)

Nose (鼻):

nas/o (nasal 鼻的), rhin/o (rhinitis 鼻炎)

Ovary (卵巢):

ovari/o (ovarian 卵巢的), oophor/o (oophorectomy 卵巢切除术)

Skin (皮肤):

cutane/o (cutaneous 皮肤的), dermat/o (dermatitis 皮炎), derm/o (dermal 真皮的), epitheli/o (epithelial 上皮的)

Uterus (子宫):

uter/o (uterine 子宫的), hyster/o (hysterectomy 子宫切除术), metri/o (endometrium 子宫内膜)

Vagina (阴道):

vagin/o (vaginal 阴道的), colp/o (colposcopy 阴道镜)

Vein (静脉):

ven/o (venous 静脉的), phleb/o (phlebitis 静脉炎)

Testes (睾丸):

orch/o (orchiectomy 睾丸切除术), orchid/o (orchidoplasty 睾丸成形术), orchi/o (orchiopexy 睾丸固定术)

Blood (血液):

hem/o (hemoglobin 血红蛋白), hemat/o (hemorrhagic 出血性的)

Colon (结肠):

col/o (colostomy 结肠造口术), colon/o (colonoscopy 结肠镜检查)

Pituitary gland (垂体):

pituitary/o (hypopituitarism 垂体功能减退), hypophys/o (hypophysis 垂体)

二、常用词根 (Common Used Roots)

词根/元音（解释）：例词

angi/o (blood vessel): angiogram 血管造影

arthr/o (joint): arthritis 关节炎

bronch/o (bronchial tube): bronchoscopy 支气管镜检查

carcin/o (cancer): carcinoma 癌

cardi/o (heart): cardiologist 心脏病学家

chron/o (time): chronic 长期的，慢性的

cephal/o (brain): cephalic 头的

cerebr/o (largest part of the brain): cerebrosclerosis 脑硬化

cervic/o (neck): cervical 子宫颈的，颈部的

col/o (large intestine): colostomy 结肠造口术

cyst/o (urinary bladder): cystitis 膀胱炎

cyt/o (cell): cytologist 细胞学家

derm/o (skin): transdermal 经皮的

dermat/o (skin): dermatologist 皮肤病医生

duoden/o (the first part of the small intestine): duodenoscope 十二指肠镜

electr/o (electricity): electrocardiogram 心电图

encephal/o (brain): encephalitis 脑炎

enter/o (intestine): gastroenterology 胃肠病学

erythr/o (red): erythrocytosis 红细胞增多症

esophag/o (food tube): esophagoscopy 食管镜检查

gastr/o (stomach): gastric 胃的

gingiv/o (gum): gingivitis 牙龈炎

glyc/o (sugar): hyperglycemia 高血糖症

gnos/o (knowledge): prognosis, diagnosis 预后、诊断

genec/o (woman): gynecologist 妇科医生

hem/o, hemat/o (blood): hemoglobin, hematoma 血红蛋白、血肿

hepat/o (liver): hepatoma 肝癌

hyster/o (uterus): hysterectomy 子宫切除

lapar/o (abdomen): laparoscope 腹腔镜

laryng/o (voice box): laryngectomy 喉头切除术

leuk/o (white): leukemia, leukocytosis 白血病、白细胞增多症

mamm/o (breast): mammogram 乳房钼靶片

mast/o (breast): mastectomy 乳房切除术

metir/o (uterus): endometrium 子宫内膜

my/o (muscle): myoma 肌瘤

nephr/o (kidney): nephrologist 肾病学家

neur/o (nerve): neuralgia 神经痛

onc/o (tumor): oncologist 肿瘤学家

oophor/o (ovary): oophorectomy 卵巢切除术

ophthalm/o (eye): ophthalmologist 眼科医师

oste/o (bone): osteomyelitis 骨髓炎

ot/o (ear): otorhinolaryngology 耳鼻喉科学

ovari/o (ovary): ovariopathy 卵巢病

path/o (disease): pathologist 病理学家

phleb/o (vein): phlebotomy 静脉切开术

pneumon/o (lung): pneumonia 肺炎

psych/o (mind): psychology 心理学

pulm/o (lung): pulmonary 肺的

radi/o (radiation): radiology 放射学

ren/o (kedney): renal 肾脏的

rhin/o (nose): rhinorrhea 流涕

sacr/o (lower back): sacral 骶骨的

sarc/o (flesh): myosarcoma 肌肉瘤

spin/o (vertebral column): spinal 脊柱的

trache/o (windpipe): tracheostomy 气管造口术

throrac/o (chest): thoracotomy 胸廓切开术

thromb/o (clotting): thrombosis 血栓形成

ur/o (urine or urea): uremia 尿毒症

vascul/o (blood vessel): vascular 血管的

第二节 前缀（Prefixes）

一、常用前缀（Common Used Prefixes）

前缀（解释）：例词

a-/an- (not): apnea, anemia 呼吸暂停，贫血

ante- (before): antenatal 产前的

anti- (against): antibiotic 抗生素，抗生素的

ab- (away from): abnormal 反常的

ad- (toward): adduct 内收

auto- (self): autopsy 尸检

brady- (slow): bradycardia 心动过缓

dia- (through/complete): diameter, diarrhea 直径，腹泻

dys- (painful/difficult): dyspnea 呼吸困难

(poor/abnormal): dysuria 排尿困难

endo- (within): endocrine glands 内分泌腺

exo- (outside): exocrine glands 外分泌腺

eu- (easy/true): eupnea 平静呼吸

hemi- (half): hemigastrectomy 半胃切除术

hyper- (excessive): hypertension 高血压

hypo- (less than normal): hypotension 低血压

macro- (very large): macroscopic 宏观的

mega- (abnormally large): megacolon 巨结肠

multi- (many): multicellular 多细胞的

peri- (surrounding): periosteum 骨膜

post- (after): postnatal 产后的

pre- (before): prenatal 产前的

pro- (before/forward): prodrome 前驱症状

re- (back): resection 切除术

retro- (behind): retroperitoneum 腹膜后

sub- (below): sublingual 舌下的

tachy- (rapid): tachycardia 心动过速

trans- (across/through): transfusion 输血

二、表方向的前缀（Prefix for Direction）

ab- (away from): abduct 外展

ad- (toward): adjacent 邻近的

dia- (through) : diameter 直径

trans- (through): transdermal 经皮的

per- (through): permeable 有渗透性的

三、表数目的前缀（Prefix for Numbers）

bi- (two): bipolar 有两极的

di- (two): diatomic 双原子的

dipl/o- (double): diplopic 复视的

hemi- (half): hemiplegia 偏瘫

mon/o- (one): monocular 单眼的

multi- (many): multicellular 多细胞的

poly- (many): polyphagia 多食症

prim/i- (first): primitive, primary 原始的，主要的

quadri- (four): quadriplegia 四肢瘫痪

semi- (half): semilunar 半月形的

tri- (three): tripod 三脚架

tetra- (four): tetrad 四分体

uni- (one): unilateral 单侧的

四、表颜色的前缀（Prefix for Colors）

cyan/o- (blue): cyanosis 发绀

erythr/o- (red): erythrocyte 红细胞

leuk/o- (white): leukoplakia 黏膜白斑

melan/o- (black, dark): melanin 黑色素

poli/o- (gray): poliomyelitis 脊髓灰质炎

xanth/o- (yellow): xanthoderma 皮肤变黄

五、表时间或位置的前缀（Prefix for Time or Position）

ante- (before): antepartum 产前的

post- (after, behind): postmortem 死后的

pre- (before, in front of): premenstrual 月经前的

pro- (before, in front of): prophase 前期

pros- (before, forward): prospective 预期的

六、表疾病的前缀（Prefix for Diseases）

brady- (slow): bradygastria 胃动过缓

dys- (abnormal): dysplasia 发育异常

　　 (difficult): dyspnea 呼吸困难

　　 (painful): dysuria 排尿困难

　　 (bad/poor): dystrophy 营养障碍

mal- (bad, poor): malignant 恶性的

pachy- (thick): pachydactyly 指（趾）肥大

staphyl/o- (grape like cluster): staphylococcus 葡萄球菌

strept/o- (twisted chain): streptobacillus 链杆菌

tachy- (fast): tachycardia 心动过速

xero- (dry): xeroma 干眼病

七、表位置或方向的前缀（Prefix for Position or Direction）

a-, an- (not, lack, without): apnea, anemia 呼吸暂停，贫血

anti- (against): antigen 抗原

circum- (around): circumcision 环切术

contra- (against): contraindicated 禁忌的

de- (down, without, removal): decongestant 减充血药

dis- (removal, separation): disinfect 给……消毒

extra- (outside): extrahepatic 肝外的

epi- (above): epidermis 表皮

infra- (below): infrascapular 肩胛下的

inter- (between): interstitial 间质的

intra- (within): intravenous 静脉内的

in-, im- (not): insignificant, impermeable 无意义的，不可渗透的

juxta- (near): juxtaposition 并列

non- (not): nonhuman 非人类的

para- (near): parathyroid gland 甲状旁腺

peri- (around): peritoneal 腹膜的

retro- (behind): retrogastric 胃后的

supra- (above): supraumbilical 脐上的

sub- (below): subpatellar 髌下的

un- (not): unconscious 无意识的

八、表程度的前缀（Prefix for Degree）

hyper- (abnormally high): hypertension 高血压

hypo- (abnormally low): hypoglycemia 低血糖症

oligo- (few): oligodontia 少牙

pan- (all): panplegia 全麻痹

super- (above): supernumerary 多余的

(excess): superscript 上标

九、表大小或比较的前缀（Prefix for Size or Comparison）

equi- (equal, same): equicaloric 等能的

eu- (true, good, easy): eupnea 平静呼吸

hemeo- (unchanging): homeostasis 内环境稳定

hetero- (different,unequal): heterosexual 异性恋的

homo- (same): homosexual 同性恋的

iso- (equal, same): isochromatic 等色的

macro- (abnormally large): macrodactyly 巨趾

mega-/megalo- (abnormally large): megacephaly 巨头畸形

micro- (small): microbiological 微生物学的

neo- (new): neocortex （大脑）新皮质

normo- (normal): normothermic 体温正常的

ortho- (straight, correct): orthopnea 端坐呼吸

poikilo- (irregular): poikilothermic 变温的

pseudo- (false): pseudogene 假基因

re- (again, back): resection 切除术

十、举例（Examples）

前缀：例词（例句）

hemi-: hemiplegia 偏瘫 (paralysis of one side of the body)

para-: paraplegia 截瘫 (condition of having lower half paralysis)

pan-: panplegia 全瘫 (condition of having total paralysis)

pseudo-: pseudoplegia 假瘫痪 (condition of having false paralysis)

quadri-: quadriplegia 四肢瘫痪 (condition of having paralysis in the four limbs)

第三节　后缀（Suffixes）

一、常用后缀（Common Used Suffixes）

后缀（解释）：例词

-al (pertaining to) : renal　肾脏的

-ac (pertaining to): cardiac　心脏的

-algia (pain): otalgia　耳痛

-algesia (pain): analgesia　痛觉缺失

-cyte (cell): erythrocyte　红细胞

-emia (blood condition): uremia　尿毒症

-globin (protein): hemoglobin　血红蛋白

-gram (record of): mammogram　乳房钼靶片

-ia (condition of): myalgia　肌痛

-ic (pertaining to): metric　公制的

-ics (medical specialty): orthopedics　整形外科

-ist (medical specialist): anesthetist　麻醉师

-ism (state of): hypothyroidism　甲状腺功能减退

-itis (inflammation): encephalitis　脑炎

-megaly (enlargment): hepatomegaly　肝大

-oma (tumor/mass): hepatoma, hematoma, nephroma　肝癌、血肿、肾瘤

-opsy (viewing): autopsy　尸检

-osis (abnormal condition of): stenosis, sclerosis　狭窄，硬化

-pathy (disease): cardiomyopathy　心肌病

-sis (state of): diagnosis　诊断

二、易混淆的后缀（Confused Suffixes）

-ectomy (excision)

Adenectomy: excision of a gland 腺切除术

-logy (study of)

Gynecology: study of women's diseases 妇科学

-logist (specialist in the study and treatment of)

Cardiologist: specialist in the study of heart 心脏病学家/医生

-scope (instrument to visually examine)

Arthroscope: an instrument to visually examine joints 关节内窥镜

-scopy (visual examination)

Ophthalmoscopy: visual examination of eyes 检眼镜检查

-stomy (+一个词根 opening to the outside of the body)

Tracheostomy: opening of the windpipe to the outside of the body 气管造口术

-stomy (+多个词根 communication)

Colocolostomy: communication between two unconnected parts of the large intestine (anastomosis) 结肠吻合术

-tome (instrument of incising)

Microtome: an instrument for cutting thin sections of tissues for microscopic study 切片机

-tomy (incision)

Laparotomy: incision into the abdomen 剖腹手术

三、举例（Examples）

-logist:

Cardiologist 心脏病医生, dermatologist 皮肤病医生, oncologist 肿瘤病医生, nephrologist 肾脏病医生, gynecologist 妇科医生, urologist 泌尿科医生, hematologist 血液病医生, biologist 生物学家, otorhinolaryngologist 耳鼻喉科医生, ophthalmologist 眼科医生, endocrinologist 内分泌科医生, gartroenterologist 消化科医生

-scopy:

Bronchoscopy 支气管镜检查，laryngoscopy 喉镜检查，laparoscopy 腹腔镜检查, gastroscopy 胃镜检查, arthroscopy 关节镜检查, cystoscopy 膀胱镜检查, ophthalmoscopy 眼底镜检查, otoscopy 耳镜检查，sigmoidoscopy 乙状结肠镜检查，rhinoscopy 鼻镜检查，uroscopy 泌尿镜检查, colonoscopy 结肠镜检查, esophagoscopy 食管镜检查

四、表专业的后缀（Suffixes for Specialties）

-ian (specialist in the field of study): optician 验光师

-iatrics (medical specialty): pediatrics 儿科学

-iatry (medical specialty): podiatry 足病学

-ics (medical specialty): obstetrics 产科学

-ist (specialist in the field of study): hematologist 血液病学家/医生

-logy (study of): neurology 神经病学

五、诊断相关的后缀（Suffixes for Diagnosis）

-gram (record of data): mammogram 乳房钼靶片

-graph (instrument for recording data): electrocardiograph 心电图仪

-graphy (act of recording data): echography 超声心动图

-meter (instrument for measuring): thermometer 温度计

-metry (measurement of): ergometry 测功

-scope (instrument for visual examination): bronchoscope 气管镜

-scopy (process of visually examining): esophagoscopy 食管镜检查

六、感官相关的后缀（Suffixes for the Senses）

-algesia (pain): analgesia 痛觉缺失

-esthesia (sensation): dysesthesia 感觉迟钝

-geusia (sense of taste): ageusia 味觉缺失

-osmia (sense of smell): parosmia 嗅觉异常

七、血液相关的后缀（Suffixes for Blood）

-emia,-hemia (condition of blood): hypoproteinemia 低蛋白血症, leucocythemia 白细胞增多症

-penia (decrease in): erythrocytopenia 红细胞减少

-poiesis (formation, production): erythropoiesis 红细胞生成

八、手术相关的后缀（Suffixes for Surgical Procedures）

-centesis (surgical puncture): thoracentesis 胸腔穿刺术

-desis (fusion): arthrodesis 关节固定术

-ectomy (excision): appendectomy 阑尾切除术

-pexy (surgical fixation): gastropexy 胃固定术

-plasty (surgical repair): rhinoplasty 鼻整形术

-rhaphy (suture): arteriorrhaphy 动脉缝合

-stomy (opening to the outside of the body): tracheostomy 气管造口术

        (communication): colocolostomy 结肠造口术

-tome (instrument to incise): microtome 显微切片机

-tomy (incision): cystotomy 膀胱切开术

-tripsy (crushing): lithotripsy 碎石术

九、药物相关的后缀（Suffixes for Drugs）

-lytic (dissolving, reducing): thrombolytic 溶栓的

-mimetic (simulating): sympathomimetic 拟交感神经的

-tropic (acting on): psychotropic 精神药物的

十、神经系统相关的后缀（Suffixes for Nervous System）

-lalia (speech): bradylalia 言语迟缓

-lepsy (seizure): narcolepsy 发作性睡病

-lexia (reading): dyslexia 阅读障碍

-mania (excited state, obsession): megalomania 狂妄自大

-paresis (partial paralysis): myoparesis 肌无力

-phasia (speech): aphasia 失语症

-phobia (irrational fear): photophobia 畏光

-plegia (paralysis): quadriplegia 四肢瘫痪

十一、视觉相关的后缀（Suffixes for Vision）

-opia (vision): diplopia 复视

-opsia (vision): achromatopsia 色盲

十二、呼吸相关的后缀（Suffixes for Respiration）

-capnia (level of carbon dioxide): eucapnia 血碳酸正常

-oxia (level of oxygen): anoxia 缺氧症

-phonia (voice): aphonia 失音症

-pnea (breathing): dyspnea 呼吸困难

十三、化学相关的后缀（Suffixes for Chemistry）

-ase (enzyme): amylase 淀粉酶

-ose (sugar): fructose 果糖

十四、疾病相关的后缀（Suffixes for Diseases）

-algia (pain): myalgia 肌痛

-algesia (pain): analgesia 痛觉缺失

-cele (hemia, localized dilation): hydrocele 鞘膜积液

-clasis, -clasia (breaking): osteoclasis 折骨术

-itis (inflammation): encephalitis 脑炎

-megaly (enlargement): cardiomegaly 心脏肥大

-odynia (pain): urodynia 排尿痛

-oma (tumor): melanoma 黑素瘤

-pathy (disease): nephropathy 肾病

-rhage, -rhagia (bursting forth, profuse flow): hemorrhage 出血,
menorrhagia 月经过多

-rhea (flow, discharge): pyorrhea 脓漏

-rhexis (rupture): hepatorrhexis 肝破裂

-schisis (splitting, fissure): thoracoschisis 胸裂畸形

十五、做后缀的疾病词语（Suffixes from Words for Diseases）

-dilation (expansion): vasodilation 血管舒张

-ectasia (distension, dilation): gastrectasia 胃扩张

-edema (swelling): papilledema 视乳头水肿

-lysis (separation, destruction, dissolving, loosening): myolysis 肌溶
血, hemolysis 溶血

-malacia (softening): craniomalacia 颅骨软化

-necrosis (death of tissue): cardionecrosis 心（肌）坏死

-ptosis (dropping): splenoptosis 脾下垂

-sclerosis (hardening): arteriosclerosis 动脉硬化

-spasm (sudden contraction): bronchospasm 支气管痉挛

-stasis (stoppage, suppression): menostasis 绝经

-stenosis (narrowing, constriction): arteriostenosis 动脉狭窄

-toxin (poison): nephrotoxin 肾毒素

第四节 拼读规则（Rules of Spelling & Pronunciation）

因拉丁语及希腊语的复杂性，本节仅介绍部分重要的拼读规则。

（1）以 rh 开头的后缀与词根连接时，r 需双写。

men(o)+rhea = menorrhea

hem(o)+rhage = hemorrhage

hemat(o)+rhagia = hematorrhagia

arteri(o)+rhaphy = arteriorrhaphy

my(o)+rhexis = myorrhexis

（2）以"x"结尾。

①"x"之前为辅音的名词，其后加后缀及变为形容词时，"x"变为"g"，如

larynx: laryngectomy, laryngeal

pharynx: pharyngotomy, pharyngeal

coccyx: coccyges, coccygeal

②"x"之前为元音的名词，其变为形容词时，"x"变为"c"，如

cervix: cervical

thorax: thoracic

（3）不规则发音。

dys[dis]: dyspnea, dysfunction

dis[dis]: dislocation

ph[f]: pharmacy

x[z]: xipoid

ch[k]: chronic

psy[si]: psychiatry

cy[si]: cytology

（4）不发音的情况。

rhinoplasty, ptosis, pneumonia, gnathic, psychiatrist, euthanasia

（5）字母"c"其后跟"i, e, y"等时常发清辅音[s], 否则发浊辅音[k]。

清辅音 [s]: cerebral, hyperglycemia, encephalogram, cytology, leukocyte, septicemia, amniocentesis, cell, incision

浊辅音 [k]: cardiology, arthroscope, cardiac, gastric, electrical, endocrinology, pericardium, medical, pharmacology

（6）字母"g"其后跟"i, e, y"等时常发清辅音[dʒ], 否则发浊辅音[g]。

清辅音 [dʒ]: hematology, enlargement, surgical, salpingitis, pharyngitis, arthralgia,angioplasty, meningitis, menorrhagia

浊辅音 [g]: hypoglycemia, electrocardiogram, organ, malignant, inguinal, mammography, ligament, gallbladder, gastric

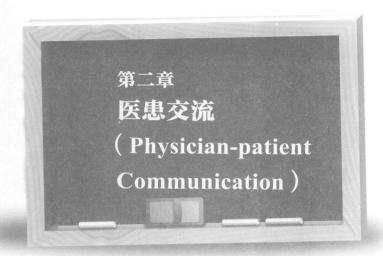

第二章
医患交流
（Physician-patient
Communication）

Declare the past,

diagnose the present,

foretell the future.

— Hippocrates

医患交流沟通的目的是有效地获取和传递信息，但患者的教育背景和理解能力参差不齐，为了避免"沟"而不"通"，无法高效地获得信息，医患交流沟通时应该采用简明易懂的词汇和语句，尽量避免深奥的专业词汇及复杂的表达方式。

本章依次介绍临床医疗活动中基本的病史采集、体格检查、辅助检查，诊疗方案、处方&用药、知情同意、手术及查房等场景中医学英语的应用。

第一节 病史采集（History Taking）

临床病史采集主要包括以下几部分内容：

Personal Details

History of Presenting Complaint

Past Medical History

Drug History

Family History

Social and Personal History

System Review

一、个人信息（Personal Details）

(1) Do you work?/ What do you do for a living?

(2) No, I'm unemployed. I'm out of work. I'm retired.

(3) Yes, I work for a bank. I'm a pensioner.

(4) Do you have a partner?

(5) Yes, I'm married. I live with my partner/spouse/husband/wife.

(6) No, I'm single/separated/divorced. I'm a widow/ widower/ divorcee.

(7) My spouse passed away last year.

二、现病史（History of Present Complaints）

现病史的采集主要围绕患者此次就诊的主要问题进行。病史采集过程中对主要症状及其相关信息的收集非常重要，尤其需注意此过程中常用动词搭配的使用，以及对症状性质、起病、持续时间、部位、严重程度、诱因及缓解因素、重要伴随症状（阴性症状）等的询问方式。

（一）常用动词（Verbs）

(1) bring on (cause, induce): is there anything special that brings on the pain?

(2) bring up (expectorate, vomit): when you cough, do you bring up any phlegm (sputum)?

(3) carry on (continue): carry on taking the painkillers for another week.

(4) come on (commence): when does the pain come on?

(5) give up (stop): my advice is to give up smoking.

(6) put on (gain weight): I've put on a lot of weight in the last months or so.

(7) turn out (happen in the end): she had all the tests and it turned out to be cancer.

(8) turn up (appear unexpectedly): the rash just turned up out of nowhere.

（二）句型（Sentence）

(1) Can you tell me what your symptoms are?

(2) Did it start suddenly (Did your condition change without any warning)?

(3) Have you ever had these complaints before?

(4) What are your symptoms (What do you think causes of your problem)?

(5) What brings it on (Can you describe the changes that have occurred)?

(6) What brings you here today?

(7) What can I do for you today (How can I help you, Mr. Braun)?

(8) When did you first notice the symptoms?

(9) When did you start feeling poorly (to fell ill)?

(10) What do you mean by that (Can you describe that in more detail)?

(11) What seems to bring this condition on?

（三）症状（Symptoms）

1. 疼痛（Pain）

疼痛是重要的临床症状之一，掌握好描述疼痛的各种形容词有助于疼痛性质的判断。下面以疼痛为例，详细举例症状病史采集中常用的词汇及句型。

1）词汇（Vocabulary）

aching/an ache: a general pain, often in muscles and joints

boring: like a drill

burning: with heat

colicky: an intermittent pain which varies in intensity, comes and goes in waves

crampy/cramp: an involuntary spasmodic muscle contraction

crushing: a feeling of pressure

dull: a background pain, opposite of sharp

gnawing: biting

gripping: a feeling of tightness

scalding: like boiling water

sharp: acute

stabbing: like a knife

stinging: sharp, burning, like an insect sting

throbbing: with a pulse or beat

2）句型（Sentences）

（1）性质（Character）

① Can you describe the pain?

② Could you please describe what the pain feels like?

③ Do you have a/an splitting (throbbing, band-like, dull, aching, burning, sharp, stabbing, colicky, migraine, blinding, stress-induced, tension) headache?

④ How bad is the pain?

⑤ Is it getting more or less severe?

⑥ Is the pain better or worse now?

⑦ What's the pain like?

⑧ What kind of pain do you feel?

⑨ What kind of pain is it?

（2）程度（Severity）

① Does it affect your work?

② Does it interfere with your everyday life?

③ Does it wake you up at night?

④ On a scale of 1 to 10 (10 being the worst), how bad is it?

⑤ On a scale of 1 to 10, with 10 being the worst pain, where would you rate your pain?

（3）起病（Onset）

① Did it happen suddenly or gradually?

② Do you have it all the time or does it seem to come and go?

③ Have you had anything like this before?

④ When does it come, and when does it go?

⑤ When did this pain start?

⑥ What were you doing at the time this pain started?

⑦ When was the last time you were without pain?

⑧ When was the first time you noticed that something was wrong?

（4）时程（Duration）

① How long have you had this pain?

② How long has it been bothering you?

③ How long does it last?

④ How often do you get it?

⑤ Is it constant or intermittent?

⑥ Is there any particular time of the day when you have the headache?

⑦ When did the headache start?

（5）部位（Location）

① Can you point with your finger to the spot where it hurts?

② Can you point out the painful area?

③ Can you show me where it hurts?

④ Does the pain seem to be coming from your neck?

⑤ Do you feel the pain at the top of your head?

⑥ Do you feel any pain in your temples (in your forehead, around your ears)?

⑦ Is the pain around your eyes (at the back of your head)?

⑧ Where does it hurt?

⑨ Where is your pain?

⑩ Where is it sore?

⑪ Whereabouts in your head is the pain?

（6）放射（Radiation）

① Does the pain move to another part of your body?

② Does the pain seem to move anywhere else (your face)?

③ Does the pain spread to your neck?

④ Does the pain travel to your shoulder?

⑤ Has the pain affected any other part of your body?

⑥ Has the pain spread?

⑥ Is the pain spreading from one to both sides of your head?

⑧ In which direction does the pain go?

（7）缓解及诱发因素（Relieving and Triggering Factors）

① After you take the medicine, how long is it before you feel better?

② Does anything relieve the symptoms or make them worse?

③ Do you take any medicine to treat the headache?

④ Have you ever blacked out?

⑤ Have you received any drugs for you pain?

⑥ How long does it take for the medicine to take effect?

⑦ Is there anything that makes it better or worse?

⑧ Is there any position that makes it feel better or worse?

⑨ Is there anything in particular that brings the pain on?

⑩ Is there anything that seems to trigger the headache?

⑪ What do you do to get rid of the headache?

⑫ What do you do when it happens?

⑬ (13) What makes the pain go away (disappear)?

（8）伴随症状（Associated Symptoms）

① Does anything else happen at the same time?

② Is it related to eating (coughing, your mood, tiredness, broken skin, body position, movement)?

③ What brings it on?

④ What are your symptoms? Is there any other symptoms accompanied with this?

3）头痛（Headache）

（1）句型（Sentences）

① Location : Show me where it hurts. Can you point out the painful area? Where does it hurt?

② Radiation: Does it go anywhere else?

③ Character: Can you describe the nature (character) of the pain?

④ Precipitating factors: Does anything bring it on?

⑤ Time of onset: When does it start?

⑥ Time of resolution: When does it stop?

⑦ Frequency: How often do you get it?

⑧ Aggravating factors: Does anything make it worse? Is there anything else that affects it? What do you do when you get the headache?

⑨ Relieving factors: Does anything make it better? Have you found any medicine that seems to help?

⑩ Duration: How long does the headache last when you get it?

⑪ Severity: On a scale of 1 to 10, 10 being the worst, how bad is it?

⑫ Associated symptoms: Do you feel anything else wrong when it's there? Do you have any other problems related to the pain? When you get the headache, does anything happen at the same time?

⑬ Family history: Does anybody else in your family has this type of headache?

（2）对话示例（Dialogue）

Physician: Tell me about your headache.

Mr. Braun: It comes and goes.

Physician: Can you point out the painful area?

Mr. Braun: It seems to be on the right side of my head.

Physician: How long does the headache last when you get it (it comes)?

Mr. Braun: It varies, it can be between half an hour and four or five hours.

Physician: When you get the headache, does anything happen at the same time?

Mr. Braun: Yeah, I often fell sick (I often feel nauseous. Sometimes I actually vomit/throw up).

Physician: Does the headache ever upset your eyes, for example, does your vision get blurred?

Mr. Braun: It's not blurry, but I get flashing lights that seem to be in the right eye.

Physician: What do you do when you get the headache?

Mr. Braun: Well, I'm not usually able to carry on with what I'm doing (I usually have to stop whatever I'm doing. I have to go to a dark room and lie down).

Physician: Have you found any tablets (medication) that seem (s) to have helped?

Mr. Braun: Sometimes if I take an aspirin early on, it seems to help. At other times nothing seems to help much.

Physician: Does anybody else in your family has this type of headache?

Mr. Braun: Yes, my mother used to suffer from migraines when she was younger.

Physician: Can you describe the character of the pain? Is it stabbing or more band-like kind of pressing?

Mr. Braun: It throbs, sort of stabbing, I suppose (I guess).

...

4）胸痛（Chest Pain）

（1）句型（Sentences）

① Do you have a burning (constricting, bursting, choking, squeezing, gripping, pressing, crushing, sticking, jabbing, sharp, sensitive, knife-like, fleeting, throbbing, dull, severe, stabbing) pain in your chest?

② Do you ever feel sweaty when this happens?

③ Have you ever had any heart problems?

④ Have you had any swelling in your feet or ankles?

⑤ Is the pain in your chest like weight on it (like a band across it)?

⑥ What seems to be the problem with your heart ?

⑦ What kind of pain do you get during exercise?

⑧ Where does the pain move?

（2）对话示例（Dialogue）

Physician: Do you feel any pain?

Mr. Braun: Yes, quite a bit.

Physician: Could you show me where it hurts?

Mr. Braun: Right here, Doctor, in my chest.

Physician: Here, hm..., is it always just in that spot?

Mr. Braun: No, sometimes it moves around to here.

Physician: I see, what kind of pain is it? Can you describe the pain?

Mr. Braun: Well, most of the time it feels like a cramp, but occasionally it's sharp and stabbing.

Physician: Does it come and go or do you have it all the time?

Mr. Braun: Well, it's worse at times. It seems to come over me in waves, but mostly it's there all the time.

Physician: Does it start suddenly or build up slowly?

Mr. Braun: It seems to build up gradually.

Physician: What do you do when you get (feel) the pain?

Mr. Braun: Well, there isn't much I can do. I just have to put up with it.

Physician: And does anything in particular seem to bring the pain on or make it worse?

Mr. Braun: Well, I find going upstairs difficult (It's more intense when climbing stairs). Also, when I have a cough or take a deep breath.

It's terrible, like a knife stabbing me.

...

5）腹痛（Abdominal Pain）

（1）句型（Sentences）

① Do you feel any/a sharp (dull, aching, gnawing, burning, cramping, colicky, diffused, localized, recurrent, constant, flank, intermittent, stabbing) pain in your abdomen?

② Do you get (feel) bloated?

③ Do you have any heartburn (indigestion)?

6）腰痛（Flank Pain）

（1）句型（Sentences）

① Do you have a sharp (dull, severe, burning, stinging, nagging, niggling, splitting, flank, back, abdominal, steady, low grade, slight) pain(ache, discomfort)?

② Do you have any problem with pissing?

③ Is your pain in the flank or lower back?

7）背痛（Back Pain）

（1）句型（Sentences）

Is the pain in your back slow in onset (long in duration, dull, diffused, aching, steady, constant, severe, progressing poorly, localized, crushing, deep, mild)?

8）肢体疼痛（Extremities）

（1）句型（Sentences）

① Do you have a/an cramp (sharp, tingling, shooting, dull, burning, severe, pulsating, throbbing) pain in your shoulder (hand, foot)?

② Do you have an ache in your hand?

③ Do you have cramp?

④ Do you have weakness (numbness, tension) in your hands (arms)?

9）牙痛（Toothache）

（1）句型（Sentences）

① Do you have a sharp (dull, throbbing, stabbing, pulsating) toothache?

② Is your toothache…?

③ Is your tooth sensitive (aching, tender, cramping)?

2. 发热（Fever）

1）词汇（Vocabulary）

extremely high, excessive perspiration, high fever, shivering, soaking wet, swinging temperature, under the tongue

2）句型（Sentences）

(1) Do you also have shivers (Do you also have chills)?

(2) Does your temperature go up and down suddenly (Are there any swings in temperature)?

(3) Do you sweat a lot (Do you perspire a lot)?

(4) Did you take your temperature under your tongue (Did you take your temperature orally)?

(5) Have you got a temperature (Have you had any fever recently? Are you feeling feverish)?

(6) Have you been abroad (Have you traveled to any countries)?

(7) I'm afraid your son's temperature is 39.5℃ (I'm sorry, but your son has an extremely high fever).

(8) I'm glad to say that your fever has fallen (You will be pleased to know that your temperature has gone down).

(9) Is your temperature high all the time (Is your temperature constantly)?

(10) I took my temperature under my tongue (I measured it orally).

(11) My entire body was shaking (My whole body was trembling).

(12) When you have a fever, do your teeth chatter (When you have a high temperature, do your teeth rattle)?

3）对话示例（Dialogue）

Physician: Have you got a temperature (had any fever recently)?

Mr. Braun: Yes, Doctor, I've been feeling quite flushed (warm) lately.

Physician: Is your temperature high all the time (constantly high) or does it go up and down?

Mr. Braun: It usually goes up at night, but it's still high even during the day (It's usually higher at night but it's still high during the day).

Physician: What is the highest and the lowest it has been in the past few days?

Mr. Braun: The highest was 39.0 °C, and the lowest was 38.0 °C.

Physician: And where did you take your temperature: under your arm or under your tongue (orally)?

Mr. Braun: I took it under my tongue (I measured it orally).

Physician: Do you also have shivers (chills)?

Mr. Braun: Yes, sometimes.

Physician: Do your teeth rattle or are the shivers (chills) milder than that?

Mr. Braun: Oh yes, they rattle. I've bitten my tongue several times already.

Physician: Do you take anything for the fever?

Mr. Braun: Aspirin.

Physician: Does it help?

Mr. Braun: No, not really.

Physician: Have you been abroad (Have you traveled) to any tropical countries recently?

Mr. Braun: Yes, I just came back from Thailand a few months ago.

Physician: I see, do you perspire more than usual?

Mr. Braun: Yes, a lot, I'm afraid.

Physician: Just when you work hard or also at other times?

Mr. Braun: Well, I never used to sweat much, but now I seem to break out in a sweat at the drop of a hat (easily). My clothes often get soaking wet.

Physician: Do you feel shaky or weak at all?

Mr. Braun: Yes, practically all the time.

...

3. 恶心&呕吐（Nausea & Vomiting）

1）词汇（Vocabulary）

belch, bring up, burp, difficult to keep anything down, feel nauseous, feeling queasy, feel sick, few spots of red blood, keep retching, little clots of blood, looks like ground coffee, projectile, spurt out in a stream, throw up, undigested food

2）句型（Sentences）

(1) Do you vomit every day (early in the morning, during the night)?

(2) Does the vomit contain undigested food (mucus, blood)?

(3) He brings up something more like bile (undigested food).

(4) I belch a lot.

(5) I feel only nauseous.

(6) It seems to be a yellowish green color.

(7) It's worse after eating (It's not related to meals).

(8) Is your vomiting related to meals (spontaneous, self-induced)?

(9) Is your nausea caused by certain places (stress, fear or depression, car or motion sickness)?

(10) Is it difficult to keep food down (bring anything up, keep liquid

down)?

(11) What you bring up, does it have a strange odor (any particular smell)?

3）对话示例（Dialogue）

Physician: Do you just feel sick (nauseous) or have you actually vomited (thrown up)?

Mr. Braun: Oh, I'm vomiting (throwing up), it seems, all the time.

Physician: When did it all start?

Mr. Braun: About two months ago.

Physician: And how often does this happen?

Mr. Braun: About once a day, sometimes more.

Physician: When are you sick? In the morning or after you have eaten?

Mr. Braun: Well, it isn't really regular.

Physician: But does it get better or worse if you eat something?

Mr. Braun: Worse, I think.

Physician: When you vomit, do you bring up digested food, undigested food or bile?

Mr. Braun: Oh, it's usually more like bile.

Physician: What color is it? Green, black, yellow or red?

Mr. Braun: It seems to be a sort of yellowish green color.

Physician: Does it ever have blood in it, or look like ground coffee?

Mr. Braun: No, never.

Physician: Do you belch (burp) a lot or have a bad (nasty) taste in your mouth?

Mr. Braun: Well, yes, Doctor, I do belch a lot and I seem to suffer from a lot of wind just lately (I have had a lot of gas lately).

...

4. 呼吸困难（Dyspnea）

1）词汇（Vocabulary）

at rest, breath in/out, during expiration/inspiration, in an horizontal position, in an upright position, lie in a lateral position, on exertion, relive, short of breath

2）句型（Sentences）

(1) Are you short of breath when you are resting or only when you are working?

(2) Can you lie flat in bed?

(3) Can you sleep on your back?

(4) Do you ever wake up at night because you are short of breath?

(5) Do you have to stop frequently when you climb the stairs?

(6) Do you feel short of breath (Do you often experience dyspnea)?

(7) Do you feel better if you take something to open your lungs (relieve the congestion) (Are your symptoms relieved by bronchodilators)?

(8) Do you feel better when you stop moving around (Does cessation of exercise relieve the dyspnea)?

(9) Do your symptoms get worse with dust or cigarettes (Is the dyspnea aggravated by dust or smoke)?

(10) Do you have to use any pillows or can you lie flat in bed (Do you need to rest in a reclined position or are you able to remain horizontal)?

(11) Does anybody in your family have any respiratory problems (Is there a history of pulmonary disease in your family)?

(12) Do you have to sit up (stand up, lie in a lateral position) when you wake up at night?

(13) How long have you had difficulty breathing?

(14) How long have you been short of breath?

(15) I usually get up and walk around when it happens.

(16) Is it relived by sitting up in bed?

(17) Is your sleep disturbed?

(18) When is your breathing most difficult?

(19) Which is more difficult, breathing in or breathing out?

(20) What do you do then?

3）对话示例（Dialogue）

示例 1

Physician: How long have you had difficulty breathing?

Mr. Braun: Since last week, Doctor.

Physician: Is it very bad?

Mr. Braun: Yes, I feel as if I can't get enough air.

Physician: Which is more difficult (what's harder), breathing in or out?

Mr. Braun: It's harder to breathe in.

Physician: Are you short of breath when you are resting or only when you are doing something (physical)?

Mr. Braun: A little when I'm resting, but it's worse when I try to do anything (physical).

Physician: Can you lie flat in bed?

Mr. Braun: No.

Physician: How many pillows do you use?

Mr. Braun: Three.

Physician: Do you ever wake up at night feeling short of breath?

Mr. Braun: Yes, I do. It frightens (scares) me because I wake up feeling as if I can't breathe.

Physician: What do you do when this happens? I mean, do you sit or stand up, does some movement help (you breathe easier)?

Mr. Braun: If I sit up, it helps a little.

Physician: Let me listen to your chest...I can hear a few crackles and it sounds a bit wheezy.

...

示例 2

Physician: What seems to be the problem at the moment (Can you tell me, what are your complaints)?

Mr. Braun: I seem to be getting very short of breath nowadays (lately), so I thought it's best to come to see you. I also feel a tightness and pain in my chest (Also I feel tightness and pain in my chest, so I thought it would be wise to come in and see you).

Physician: How long has this been going on?

Mr. Braun: It seems to have been getting worse over the last few weeks.

Physician: Are you short of breath all the time, or is it just when you walk up the stairs (exert yourself)?

Mr. Braun: Well, it's hard work going up the stairs. The pain feels like stabbing (Well, the pain gets worse when I exert myself. It fells like stabbing).

Physician: Does the pain move (radiate) to other areas as well?

Mr. Braun: Yes, it moves (radiates) to my neck, my left arm, my back and my left shoulder.

Physician: Do you ever feel sick or sweaty when that happens?

Mr. Braun: Well, I don't feel sick but I often break out in (to) a sweat.

Physician: Do you ever feel that your heart beats unusually fast or slow?

Mr. Braun: Yes, sometimes it beats really slowly. Then from time to time it skips a beat, then continues to beat very rapidly.

Physician: Can you tap out with a finger what the rhythm feels like to you... Good. Have you had any swelling in your ankles?

Mr. Braun: Yes, both of my feet have been somewhat swollen.

Physician: Does it go down overnight or are they still swollen in the morning?

Mr. Braun: Oh, my feet feel much better, and they aren't as swollen in the morning.

5. 抑郁（Depression）

1）句型（Sentences）

(1) Do you find you wake up very early in the morning?

(2) Have you been feeling sad, down or blue?

(3) Have you felt depressed or lost interest in things daily for two or more weeks in the past?

(4) Have you ever felt like taking your own life (risk of self-harm)?

(5) Has your appetite been poor recently?

(6) Have you lost weight recently?

(7) How do you feel about the future?

(8) Have you had trouble concentrating on things?

(9) Have you had guilty thoughts?

(10) Have you lost interest in things you usually enjoy?

6. 焦虑（Anxiety）

1）句型（Sentences）

(1) Do you feel suddenly frightened, or anxious or panicky, for no reason in situations in which most people would not be afraid?

(2) Do you find you have to do things repetitively, such as washing your hands multiple times?

(3) Do you feel uncomfortable in crowded places?

(4) Do you have trouble relaxing?

(5) Do you have problems getting to sleep at night?

(6) Do you have any rituals (such as checking things) that you feel you have to do, even though you know it may be silly?

(7) Do you have recurrent thoughts that you have trouble controlling?

(8) Do you worry excessively about things?

(9) Do you worry excessively about minor things?

2）对话示例（Dialogue）

Physician: What seems to be the problem at the moment?

Mr. Braun: Well, I've been feeling so poorly recently (ill lately).

Physician: I see. Feeling poorly. What do you mean by that?

Mr. Braun: I've been getting (I've been) very short of breath.

Physician: Hm.... how long has this been going on?

Mr. Braun: For about 5 months, I think.

Physician: And were there any other symptoms before then or did it start quite suddenly?

Mr. Braun: I hadn't noticed anything before then.

Physician: So you haven't experienced this symptom before (So you didn't have any of these symptoms before)?

Mr. Braun: No, not that I can remember, Doctor.

Physician: I see. Was there anything that seemed to cause this?

Mr. Braun: Well, nothing, really. Except maybe it gets really bad when I go to see my sister.

Physician: Let's take a look (to begin with). I'll listen to your heart and lungs to begin with.

7. 患者关注/期望（Patient Attention & Expectations）

(1) Do you have any ideas about this?

(2) Do you have any concerns?

(3) How do you think you get this problem?

(4) How might this affect the rest of your family?

(5) What are your worries about?

(6) What do you think will happen?

(7) What do you expect from me?

(8) What do you mean by...?

(9) What do you know about this problem/condition/illness?

(10) What are you hoping we could do for you?

三、既往史（Past Medical History）

1. 句型（Sentences）

(1) Are your parents still alive?

(2) Are you currently taking any medicine?

(3) Have you ever seen double?

(4) Did you have any childhood disease?

(5) Do you have any problems with your teeth?

(6) Have you ever had an operation (a blood transfusion)?

(7) Have you ever been in the hospital?

(8) Have you had your vaccinations?

(9) What kind of treatment do you receive?

2. 对话示例（Dialogue）

Physician: I'd like to ask you about your past medical history. Can you tell me whether you have had any childhood diseases, for example chickenpox, measles, mumps or German measles?

Mr. Braun: When I was small, I had measles, chickenpox and whooping cough, but I don't think I ever had German measles /rubella.

Physician: Have you ever been in hospital (hospitalized) for anything? Or have you ever had an operation?

Mr. Braun: Well, I had my tonsils taken/ out when I was a child.

Physician: Have you had any major health problems since then?

Mr. Braun: Yes, I have diabetes.

Physician: When were you first told that you had (diagnosed with) diabetes? What were your symptoms?

Mr. Braun: After I was 14 (I was diagnosed when I turned 14). I was always thirsty, tired and depressed.

Physician: Are you receiving any treatment for your diabetes (this)?

Mr. Braun: I've been having (getting) insulin (shots) ever since.

Physician: Are you up to date with all your immunizations?

Mr. Braun:Yes.

Physician: Good. Let me have a look at the letter from your general physician. (Did your referring physician give you a letter for me?)

Mr. Braun: Yes, here it is.

...

四、用药史（Drug History）

包括 name, dose, indication, frequency, allergy, drug reaction 等。

1. 句型（Sentences）

(1) Are you taking any medication at the moment?

(2) Do you actually take all of the regular medications prescribed for you?

(3) Do you always remember to take it?

(4) Do you get any side effects?

(5) Do you know if you are allergic to any drug (what symptoms do you get after taking it)?

(6) Do you take any recreational drugs?

(7) Do you use any over-the-counter remedies or herbal or homeopathic medicines?

(8) How many times a day?

(9) Have you recently changed, started or stopped any medications?

(10) Which tablet do you take?

五、家族史（Family History）

1. 句型（Sentences）

(1) Are all your close relatives alive?

(2) Are your parents alive and well?

(3) Are there any illnesses that run in the family?

(4) Are there any medical problems with your kids (Is there anything wrong with your children's health)?

(5) At what age did your father die (how old was your dad when he passed away)?

(6) And your aunt who has diabetes, does she still have a weight problem?

(7) Do you have any brothers or sisters?

(8) Do you have any children?

(9) Do you know the cause of death?

(10) Does anyone in your family have a serious illness?

(11) How did your father die?

(12) How is your aunt's health?

(13) How old was he when he died?

(14) Is anyone taking regular medication?

(15) Is there anyone in your family who suffers from mental illness?

(16) What did he die of?

2. 对话示例（Dialogue）

Physician: As far as you know, are there any illnesses that run in your family?

Mr. Braun: None (Not) that I know of, Doctor.

Physician: Nothing like diabetes, high blood pressure, or heart disease, stroke, cancer, mental illness or anything like that?

Mr. Braun: Oh, I see! My father had a heart condition, and I have two aunts who have diabetes.

Physician: And is your father still alive?

Mr. Braun: No, he isn't.

Physician: How old was your father when he died (passed away)?

Mr. Braun: He was 66.

Physician: What did he die of?

Mr. Braun: He had a heart attack.

Physician: Did he suffer for a long time with his heart condition before he died (Did he have an ongoing heart condition)?

Mr. Braun: Oh no, it was very sudden.

Physician: And your aunts? Do you know what kind of diabetes they have? Are your aunts taking any medications right now for their diabetes [Do they have to take insulin (shots) or tablets (oral medications), or are they just on a diet]?

Mr. Braun: They just take some pills, I think.

Physician: You are married, I see. Do you have any children?

Mr. Braun: Yes, a boy and a girl.

Physician: Are they healthy?

Mr. Braun: Yes, they are.

六、社会及个人史(Social and Personal History)

1. 句型（Sentences）

(1) Are any of them at nursery or school?

(2) Are you aware of any difference in your alcohol consumption

over the past five years?

(3) Can you give up alcohol when you want?

(4) Do you live alone?

(5) Do you smoke?

(6) Do you have any problems at work?

(7) Do you have any financial problems?

(8) Do you have any hobbies or interests?

(9) How many (do you smoke) a day?

(10) How much do you drink weekly?

(11) How old are your children?

(12) Have you tried giving up?

(13) What about alcohol? Wine, beer or spirits?

(14) What about exercise?

(15) What's the most you would drink in a week?

(16) What kind of house do you live in?

(17) Who shares your home with you?

(18) What's your occupation?

2. 对话示例（Dialogue）

Physician: Do you have a job at the moment (Are you working right now)?

Mr. Braun: No, I've just been made redundant (laid off).

Physician: Oh, I am sorry. What was your job?

Mr. Braun: I was a civil servant in Customs and Excise (I was a manager in an import and export company).

Physician: I see. Was it an office job or were you on your feet all day?

Mr. Braun: I was desk-bound, I'm afraid (I worked behind a desk).

Physician: Was it managerial — did you have a lot of responsibility?

Mr. Braun: Yes, I was in charge of a large department.

Physician: I see, quite stressful. Now tell me, sir, do you smoke?

Mr. Braun: Yes, I do (Unfortunately, quite a bit).

Physician: Oh, really, how much?

Mr. Braun: Oh, about forty (two packs) a day.

Physician: How long have you been smoking?

Mr. Braun: Since I was about ten.

Physician: Have you ever tried to give up (quit) smoking?

Mr. Braun: Yes, I've tried to give it up several times, but without success.

Physician: What about drinking? Do you drink?

Mr. Braun: Yes, sometimes with my friends.

Physician: How much alcohol do you drink a day?

Mr. Braun: Let's see. A couple of pints in the pub (glasses of beer) at lunch time, a whisky in the evening and about half a bottle of wine with our meal (my dinner).

Physician: That's quite a bit. How old were you when you started drinking?

Mr. Braun: Oh, about 18, I suppose.

Physician: What sort of house do you live in (what about your living conditions? Where do you live)?

Mr. Braun: We live in a small flat (apartment). It's our own but we are still paying the mortgage on it, of course (We own it, but of course we are still paying the mortgage on it).

...

七、系统回顾（System Review）

1. 句型（Sentences）

(1) Any burning or stinging sensation?

(2) Do you bring up anything and what color is it?

(3) Do you ever have any difficulty breathing?

(4) Do you ever have any chest pain?

(5) Do you ever experience palpitations?

(6) Do you ever have any problems passing water?

(7) Do you have a cough?

(8) Do you have any problems with your joints?

(9) Do you have any problems with your ears, nose or throat?

(10) Have you ever had any fits, faints or funny turns?

(11) Have you had any changes in your bowel habit? Any changes to the stool? Increased frequency?

(12) Have you had any fevers or night sweats?

(13) Have you developed any rashes?

(14) Has there been any unintentional weight loss?

(15) Pass a lot of water? When did this start?

2. 心血管系统（Cardiovascular System）

(1) Are you short of breath on exertion? How much exertion is necessary?

(2) Can you lie flat without feeling breathless?

(3) Do you have cold or blue hands or feet?

(4) Do you have pain in your legs on exercise?

(5) Have you ever had rheumatic fever, a heart attack or high blood pressure?

(6) Have you ever woken up at night short of breath? (Heart failure)

(7) Have you felt dizzy or blacked out when exercising? (Severe aortic stenosis or hypertrophic cardiomyopathy)

(8) Have you had any pain or pressure in your chest, neck or arm? (Myocardial ischemia)

(9) Have you had swelling of your ankles?

(10) Have you noticed your heart racing or beating irregularly?

(11) Have you had blackouts without warning? (Stokes-Adams attacks)

3. 呼吸系统（Respiratory System）

(1) Are you ever short of breath? Has this come on suddenly? (Pulmonary embolism)

(2) Do you cough up anything?

(3) Do you ever have wheezing when you are short of breath?

(4) Do you have night sweats?

(5) Do you snore loudly? Do you fall asleep easily during the day? When? Have you fallen asleep while driving? (Obtain a sleep history)

(6) Have you coughed up blood? (Bronchial carcinoma)

(7) Have you ever had pneumonia or tuberculosis?

(8) Have you had a recent chest X-ray?

(9) Have you had fevers?

(10) Have you had any cough?

(11) Is your cough associated with shivers, shakes (rigors), breathlessness or chest pain? (Pneumonia)

(12) What type of work have you done? (Occupational lung disease)

4. 消化系统（Gastrointestinal System）

(1) Are you troubled by indigestion? What do you mean by indigestion?

(2) Do you have heartburn?

(3) Have you had any difficulty swallowing? (Esophageal cancer)

(4) Have you had vomiting, or vomited blood? (Gastrointestinal bleeding)

(5) Have you had pain or discomfort in your abdomen?

(6) Have you had any abdominal bloating or distension?

(7) Has your bowel habit changed recently? (Carcinoma of the colon)

(8) How many bowel motions a week do you usually pass?

(9) Have you lost control of your bowels or had accidents (fecal incontinence)?

(10) Have you seen blood in your motions? (Gastrointestinal bleeding)

(11) Have your bowel motions been black? (Gastrointestinal bleeding)

(12) Have you lost weight recently without dieting? (Carcinoma of the colon)

(13) Have your eyes or skin ever been yellow?

(14) Have you ever had hepatitis, peptic ulceration, colitis or bowel cancer?

(15) Tell me (briefly) about your diet recently.

5. 内分泌系统（Endocrine System）

(1) Do your hands tremble?

(2) Do you prefer hot or cold weather?

(3) Have you noticed any swelling in your neck?

(4) Have you had a thyroid problem or diabetes?

(5) Have you noticed increased sweating?

(6) Have you been troubled by fatigue?

(7) Have you noticed any change in your appearance, hair, skin or voice?

(8) Have you been unusually thirsty lately? Or lost weight? (New onset of diabetes)

6. 血液系统（Hematological System）

(1) Do you bruise easily?

(2) Do you have difficulty in stopping a small cut from bleeding? (Bleeding disorder)

(3) Have you had fevers, or shivers and shakes (rigors)?

(4) Have you noticed any lumps under your arms, or in your neck or groin? (Hematological malignancy)

(5) Have you ever had blood clots in your legs or in the lungs?

7. 神经系统及意识状态（Neurological System and Mental State）

(1) Are you dizzy?

(2) Do you get headaches?

(3) Do you have trouble seeing or hearing?

(4) Do you feel sad or depressed, or have problems with your "nerves"?

(5) Do you get ringing in the ears?

(6) Have you had fainting episodes, fits or blackouts?

(7) Have you had weakness, numbness or clumsiness in your arms or legs?

(8) Have you ever had a stroke or head injury?

(9) Have you had difficulty sleeping?

(10) Have you ever been sexually or physically abused?

(11) Have you ever experienced any numbness or tingling in your hands or feet?

(12) Have you ever had a blackout?

(13) Is your headache very severe and did it begin very suddenly? (Subarachnoid hemorrhage)

8. 肌肉骨骼系统（Musculoskeletal System）

(1) Are any of your joints red, swollen and painful?

(2) Do you have painful or stiff joints?

(3) Do you have any back or neck pain?

(4) Do your fingers ever become painful and become white and blue in the cold?

(5) Have you had a skin rash recently?

(6) Have your eyes been dry or red?

(7) Have you ever had a dry mouth or mouth ulcers?

(8) Have you been diagnosed as having rheumatoid arthritis or gout?

9. 生殖泌尿系统（Genitourinary System）

(1) Are you passing larger or smaller amounts of urine?

(2) Are your periods regular?

(3) Do you have difficulty or pain in passing urine?

(4) Do you have to get up at night to pass urine?

(5) Do you have excessive pain or bleeding with your periods?

(6) Do you have any problems with your sex life? Difficulty obtaining or maintaining an erection?

(7) Has the urine colour changed?

(8) Have you seen blood in your urine? (Urinary tract malignancy)

(9) Have you noticed any rashes or lumps on your genitals?

(10) Have you ever had a sexually transmitted disease?

(11) Have you ever had a urinary tract infection or kidney stone?

(12) Is your urine stream as good as it used to be?

(13) Is there a delay before you start to pass urine? (Applies mostly to men)

(14) Is there dribbling at the end?

10. 女性月经生育史（Menstrual & Reproductive History）

(1) Are your periods very painful?

(2) Are you using any kind of contraception?

(3) Could you tell me when your first/last period was?

(4) Do you have a regular cycle?

(5) Do you get any bleeding in between your periods?

(6) Do you find you are using a lot of pads?

(7) Do you think you might be pregnant?

(8) Have you had any terminations?

(9) Have you had any miscarriages?

(10) Have you had high blood pressure or diabetes in pregnancy?

(11) Have you had a Caesarean section?

(12) Have you had any bleeding or discharge from your breasts or felt any lumps there? (Carcinoma of the breast)

(13) How long do your periods last for?

(14) How many pregnancies have you had?

(15) How many children do you have?

(16) Is the discharge foul smelling at all?

(17) Is this your first pregnancy?

(18) Were there any other complications during your pregnancies or deliveries?

(19) Would you say that your periods are quite light, average or heavy?

11. 老年患者（The Elderly Patient）

(1) Are you affected by any chronic diseases?

(2) Can you manage at home without help?

(3) Do you walk with a frame or stick?

(4) Do you take sleeping tablets or sedatives? (Fall risk)

(5) Do you take blood pressure tablets? (Postural hypotension and fall risk)

(6) Have you had problems with your memory or with managing things like paying bills? (Cognitive decline)

(7) How do you manage your various tablets? (Risk of polypharmacy and confusion of doses)

(8) Have you had problems with falls or loss of balance? (High fracture risk)

(9) Have you been tested for osteoporosis?

八、病史采集技巧（History Taking Skills）

(1) Start with open questions but finish with specific questions to narrow the differential diagnosis.

(2) Do not hurry.

(3) Ask the patient "What else?" to ensure that all problems have been identified.

(4) Maintain comfortable eye contact and an open posture. Use the head nod appropriately.

(5) When there are breaks in the narrative, provide a summary for the patient by briefly restating the facts or feelings identified, to maximize accuracy and demonstrate active listening.

(6) Clarify the chief or presenting complaints with the patient, while not assuming that you know them.

(7) If you are confused about the chronology of events or other issues, ask the patient to clarify.

(8) Make sure the patient's story is internally consistent.

(9) Show respect and sympathy.

(10) Ask about any other concerns the patient may have, and address

specific fears.

(11) Express your support and willingness to help solve the problems together.

九、老年人病史采集（History Taking in Elderly）

1. 注意之处（Special Attention）

(1) Presenting complaint: only one complaint is unusual!

(2) Past history: record the patient's immunization status, especially for pneumococcus, influenza and tetanus.

(3) Medications: many old patients will be taking multiple medications for several chronic diseases (polypharmacy). A comprehensive list including reason for use is important in terms of planning management. Pay attention to any new symptoms which may be associated with polypharmacy.

(4) Social history: accommodation, exercise, smoking, alcohol use, abuse and neglect.

(5) Review of systems: concentrate especially on vision, hearing, chewing and dentition, weight changes, fecal and urinary incontinence, recurrent falls, a history of fractures and foot disease.

2. 句型（Sentences）

(1) Are you able to walk without difficulty?

(2) Do you exercise regularly?

(3) Do you drive?

(4) Do you feel that you eat well? Do your teeth give you trouble?

(5) Do you have any trouble managing cooking, washing or banking?

(6) Do you worry that you will not be able to cope in the future? Have you thought how you will manage if your health gets worse?

(7) During the past month have you been feeling down, depressed or hopeless? During the past month, have you been bothered by little interest or pleasure in doing things?

(8) How is your vision? Have you had cataracts? Do you wear glasses?

(9) How is your hearing? Have you got hearing aids? Do they work?

(10) Have you fallen over in the past year? Do you have arthritis or Parkinson's disease?

(11) Have you had any fractures of your spine? Wrists? Hips?

(12) What do you think your main problems are at the moment?

(13) Would you allow me to talk to any of your relatives or friends about your health issues?

(14) With whom do you live?

(15) What tablets are you taking? Do you have trouble remembering to take them? Have any of your medications changed recently? Do you think they have caused you any problems?

Don't touch the patient —

state first what you see,

cultivate your powers of observation.

— William Osler

One finger in throat and one in the rectum

makes a good diagnostician.

— William Osler

体格检查是在病史采集的基础上，通过医生的"视、触、叩、听"（inspection, palpation, percussion, auscultation）等物理诊断手段，以发现可佐证患者主诉症状的阳性体征，为下一步辅助检查、诊断和鉴别诊断提供线索。在体格检查过程中，无论是全身体格检查还是重点专科体格检查，医师都会说一些祈使句和解释性话语让患者配合检查，熟悉掌握这些语句将会帮助医师顺利高效地完成体格检查。

一、常用动词组（Verbs）

bend down

breathe in/out

close your eyes

curl up

do this please

follow my fingertip with your eyes

put your head down

put out your tongue

raise your leg

keep your knee straight

let you wrist go floppy

lie on your side/back

lie on the bed/couch

lie down

open your mouth

point to the finger that moves

pull as hard as you can

push as hard as you can

roll on to your back/front

roll over

roll up your sleeve

sit, sit up

slide your hand down your side

slip off your coat

stand straight

stand up

take off your top things

tilt your head back

touch your shoulder with your chin

turn your head to the left

turn on your side

relax please

show me what movements you can manage

tell me if it hurts

二、常用表部位介词（Prepositions）

熟悉下列常见介词的用法，有利于准确地描述体格检查结果。

（1）"at"用于较局限部位和点

at the apex of the heart

at the left lower chest area

at the right angle of the mandible

The spleen tip was palpable at the left costal margin.

A few fine rales were also heard at the right base posteriorly.

（2）"in"用于较大场所和部位，若表示"在……里面"时，可用于小地方

pain in the stomach

weakness and numbness in the left hand

have aching in various joints

have a mass in the right mid-abdomen

There is one soft, fluctuating cystic mass arising from the skin in the suprapubic area.

There is a painless swelling in the roof of the mouth.

（3）"on" 用于表示与表面接触的部位

a necrotic ulcer on the tip of the tongue

on the right lower gingiva

vague headache on the left side

a painful ulcer on the left thigh

Crusted lesions were seen on all skin surfaces.

（4）"over" 用于表示其上的部位

itching on the skin over the upper back

a nodule over the right wrist

Examination of the lung fields revealed the breath sounds to be diminished over the left upper chest anteriorly and posteriorly.

（5）"above" 用于表示部位的高低，在上面 (higher than)

On admission there was a moderate degree of jaundice and a small scar above the left costal margin.

A pea-sized nodule is felt above the nipple.

（6）"beneath" 用于表示底下的接触

There is a tender swelling beneath the right buccal mucosa.

She first noticed hyperpigmentation of the skin beneath both breasts in Feb. 2020.

（7）"under" 用于表示其下的部位

Tumors are palpated under the skin.

He was examined with a 5-hour complaint of pain and swelling under the left jaw in the floor of the mouth.

（8）"below" 用于表示在下面 (lower than)

The uterus was palpated 2 finger-breadths below the umbilicus.

The patient has a radiolucent lesion below the molar teeth in the right mandible.

（9）"along" 用于表示沿一长线的部位

A systolic (grade Ⅳ) murmur radiates along the left sternal border.

A murmur was heard along the sternal border.

（10）"around" 用于表示周围静止的部位

The pain was centered around the left eye and forehead.

For three years this patient was aware of a twitching of the muscles around her left eye and a progressive left facial weakness.

三、常用句型（Sentences）

(1) Good morning, I'm Dr Huang.

(2) Do you know what we're going to do this morning?

(3) What we're going to do today is...

(4) I'm going to examine your..., so I can find out what's causing this...

(5) What we do is...

(6) What happens is that...

(7) I'll ask you to...

(8) I'll examine you now.

(9) Would you mind taking off all your clothes except your underwear (men) and bra (women)?

(10) Lie on the stretcher with your shoes and socks off, please.

(11) Roll your sleeve up, please, I'm going to examine your elbow.

(12) Are you ready?

(13) You might feel a little bit of discomfort.

(14) This might hurt a little but I'll be quick.

(15) Tell me if it hurts.

(16) Let me know if it is sore.

(17) It will be over very quickly.

(18) It won't take long.

(19) You're doing very well.

(20) I'm just going to...

(21) First (then) I'll...

(22) Now I'm going to...

(23) You'll feel...

(24) When it's over, I'll...

(25) That's it. All over.

(26) Well, I'm fairly certain you've got a ....

(27) One possibility is that it could be what we called...

(28) I haven't found anything to suggest any problems.

(29) Could you bend forward as far as you can?

(30) If you could cross your arms in front of your chest.

(31) What I'd like to do is to examine you when you keep standing up.

(32) Stand with your feet together.

(33) Lie perfectly still.

(34) Can you just turn to the side again?

(35) Could you just lie on the couch?

(36) You can get dressed now (Please get dressed). Take your time, we are not in a hurry.

四、全身体格检查（General Physical Examination）

（一）常用句型（Sentences）

(1) Good afternoon, Mr. Braun, I'm Dr. Xu, I'd like to examine you now.

(2) Will you please strip down (get undressed to waist) and put on the white gown in that room?

(3) Lie on the couch and cover yourself with the blanket.

(4) Let me check your temperature.

(5) Open your mouth. Stick your tongue out, move the tongue up and down, to the left and right.

(6) I want to check your throat. Please open your mouth wide and stick your tongue out, Say ah…

(7) Look at this finger, and follow the finger without moving your head.

(8) Follow my fingers with your eyes only.

(9) Take deep breaths. Hold the breath.

(10) Breathe quietly through your nose... over and over.

(11) Now, blow your air out and hold it.

(12) Blow out all your breath.

(13) Breathe in and out through your mouth.

(14) Now, stop breathing completely.

(15) Don't breathe now.

(16) Will you say "nine"?

(17) Say ninety-nine please.

(18) Would you turn around so that I can see your back?

(19) Will you please stand up straight with your back toward me?

(20) Please bend slightly forward. I will tap your spine. Tell me when it hurts.

(21) Does it hurt here?

(22) Did it hurt you anywhere when I touched you? Any tender spot?

(23) Turn your body from your waist.

(24) Please lie down on the table, bring your knees up, and relax your stomach. Take a deep breath. Tell me when it hurts where I press.

(25) Lie down on your back in that bed. Bend your knees, relax, don't be so stiff and tight.

(26) Take a deep breath, breathe with the belly not with the chest.

(27) Does this hurt you? Which is more painful when I press here or when I release the finger?

(28) Which hurts more, when I press down or when I release the pressure?

(29) Lie on your right side, please.

(30) Turn to your right.

(31) Face this side please.

(32) Give me your right arm, I want to check your blood pressure. Let me put the blood pressure cuff around your arm, and please relax, so your blood pressure will not go up. It's 120 over 70... Now, the left side... Your blood pressure is normal. We have to examine your urine and also take an electrocardiogram.

(33) Let me see how you walk. Walk over to the window, turn around and come back. Try to walk straight and quick.

(34) Now, please walk toward the window, faster!

(35) Please stand there with your feet together. Now close your eyes. Don't worry about falling, I will catch you.

（二）神经系统（Nervous System）

1. 句型（Sentences）

1）定向力（Orientation）

(1) Can you tell me your name and address? I'm going to ask you some simple questions to assess how good your concentration is.

(2) Can you tell me what day of the week it is today? What month are we in? What year is it?

(3) Approximately what time of the day is it at the moment? Can you

tell me anything that is going on in the news at present? What's the name of the president?

(4) I'm going to give you an imaginary name and address. And I want you to remember the name and address, and after five minutes I'll ask you to repeat the name and address to me.

(5) Now I'd like to assess how clear your speech is. Say more words for me. Start by saying the days of the week, start with Monday.

(6) Now, I'm going to ask you to say some more difficult things. Say after me " Olympic Game" "The European Commission".

(7) Now I'm going to examine your understanding of the words that I say to you.

(8) Lift your right hand in the air. Touch your right ear with the little finger of your left hand.

(9) Now I'd like to see how you walk. I want you to stand up and walk to the other side of the room, then turn around and come back to me.

2）颅神经（Cranial Nerves）

(1) Cover one nostril and smell this substance. Tell me what it smells like.

(2) I'd like to check your vision. Read the chart in front of you, please, starting from about here.

(3) I'm going to assess what you can see out of the corner of your eye. Look at the middle of my face and point at my finger when I wiggle it.

(4) Now I'm going to shine a light in your eye to look at the reactions of the pupil. Keep looking straight ahead. Keep looking straight ahead, while I shine a light in the back of your eyes to examine the retina. Try and keep looking forward at the wall behind me. Try and ignore the light.

(5) Now I'm going to assess the movements of your eyes. Hold your

head still and follow my finger just by moving your eyes.

(6) Now, I'm going to assess the feeling on your face. I'm going to touch the skin on your face very lightly with some cotton wool. Say "yes" when I touch your face and keep your eyes closed.

(7) Now I want to examine the strength in the muscles of your face. Screw your eyes up very tightly. Don't let me open them. Now purse your lips together very tightly. Stop me from opening them. Blow your cheeks out like this.

(8) Now I'm going to test your hearing. Tell me if you can hear what I'm whispering into each ear in turn: 88, 66.

(9) Now, I want to examine the muscles of the back of your mouth. Open your mouth wide, and say "ah".

(10) I'm going to test the feeling at the back of your mouth. Tell me if you feel a gentle touch of the wooden stick.

(11) Now open your mouth wide again and stick your tongue out. Wiggle your tongue quickly from side to side.

(12) Finally, shrug your shoulder against me and turn your head to one side and then turn it to the other side, so that I can see the strength of the muscles in your neck.

3）运动功能（Motor Function）

(1) Now we're moving on to examine your arms and legs neurologically.

(2) Start by putting both arms out in the air in front of you and close your eyes.

(3) Hold the arms still while I look at them. Now wiggle your fingers as if you were playing the piano.

(4) Now let me assess the coordination in your arms. Open your eyes, make a pointer by stretching out your index finger. Now touch my finger and then touch your nose. Go between my finger and your nose with your

finger very quickly. Now try this on the other side.

(5) Now I'm going to assess the strength in the muscles of your arms.

(6) Stick your arms out on both sides to show me the strength of your shoulder muscles.

(7) Now pull the elbows down towards your sides.

(8) Now testing each arm in turn, make a fist and pull the fist up towards your shoulder while I try to stop you.

(9) Now straighten your arm out at the elbow while I try to stop you. Do that again on the other side.

(10) Now holding both arms in front of you, make two fists and cock the wrists backwards. Stop me from moving the wrists. Now cock the wrists downwards, while I try to stop you. Now do the same with the fingers.

(11) Stretch all your fingers out straight and stop me from bending your fingers.

(12) Now curl your fingers up tightly into my fingers and make a strong grip. Keep the fingers tightly curled up.

(13) Now squeeze my fingers as tight as you can in both hands.

(14) Now spread your fingers wide apart while I test the small muscles in the hand. Stop me from pushing the fingers together... OK, very good.

(15) Now I'm going to examine the sensation on your skin. Keep your eyes closed throughout the examination.

(16) I'm going to touch the skin of your arms in various different places just using a light touch with cotton wool. Say "yes" every time I touch the skin.

(17) Now I'm going to test the same feeling, but using the prick of a pin instead of cotton woo. Say "yes" every time you feel the touch of the pin. Can you feel the pinprick? Does it feel the same on both sides?

(18) Now, I'm going to assess whether you can feel vibration. I'll start with your hand. Tell me if you can feel the vibration of the tuning fork.

(19) Finally, I'm going to assess whether you can feel your finger being moved up and down. I'm going to hold your little finger and move it up and down slowly. Shut your eyes and when you feel the finger move up say "up" and when it's down say "down".

(20) Now, I'm going to test the reflexes in your arms. Relax your arms and I'll tap the reflexes of the biceps and triceps muscles, and also the supinator reflex.

(21) I'm going to test the reflexes in your legs. Relax your legs while I tap the reflexes in the knees and at the ankles.

(22) I'm going to scratch the bottom of your foot with a wooden stick.

(23) I'd like to assess your walking. Let me see you walk around. Just slowly. Walk 20 or 30 feet away from me, then turn around and walk back towards me.

(24) Relax your legs while I move them around slowly. Now let me see the strength in the muscles. Lift your left leg up in the air and hold it straight. Now let me look at the other side. Now put the leg down flat onto the examination table. Now the other side.

(25) Bend the knee and keep it bent. Stop me from straightening it. Now kick the leg straight against me.

(26) Flex your foot up toward your face and stop me from pulling it down. Now push the foot away from you to push me away.

(27) Turn the foot so the sole of the foot is facing the other foot and keep it there.

(28) Now turn the sole of the foot outwards and keep it there. Stop me from straightening the ankle.

(29) I'm going to touch you with a small piece of cotton wool on the leg. Shut your eyes and say "yes" when you feel the touch of the cotton wool. I want to compare the two sides. Tell me if the touch feels the same on the left leg as it does on the right.

(30) Now I'm going to test sensation using a pinprick. Tell me whether there's a clear difference between the touch of the pin and the cotton wool.

(31) Can you feel the vibration of the tuning fork when I press it onto the bones in your ankle?

(32) I'm going to wiggle your big toe up and down. Shut your eyes and say "up" when I move the toe up, "down" when I move the toe down.

（三）精神状态（Mental Status）

1. 句型（Sentences）

(1) Can you describe your mood at the moment?

(2) Can you keep your mind on things?

(3) Do you take pleasure in anything?

(4) How are your energy levels?

(5) How long have you been feeling like this?

(6) Have you noticed any change in your weight?

(7) How is your sleeping?

(8) Have you ever felt that you don't want to go on?

(9) Have you ever thought of suicide?

(10) What's your appetite like?

(11) What do you feel the future holds for you?

（四）体格检查示例（Examples of Physical Examination）

1. 示例 1（Case 1）

Vital signs: T: 39.0 °C, P: 110 bpm, R: 24 bpm, BP: 120/82 mmHg

The patient was a talkative, alert, elderly male in no acute distress and without cyanosis.

Skin: Mild palmar erythema.

Hair: Not remarkable.

Eyes: Slightly prominent, blinking somewhat infrequently, but otherwise normal.

E.N.T: Neg. Except edentulous.

Neck: Thyroid diffusely enlarged 2-3 times more than normal without bruit.

Heart: Not enlarged. No murmurs. A2 greater than P2. Normal sinus rhythm.

Lungs: Trachea in midline. Percussion note hypersesonat and breath sounds distant throughout. There were a few sticky rales at both lung bases; no rubs were heard.

Abdomen: Protuberant. Liver descends 3 f.b. from the right costal margin following inspiration.

Spleen: Not palpable. Moderate right upper quadrant and epigastric tenderness.

Genitalia: Normal.

Rectal: Grade Ⅱ hypertrophy of prostate.

Extremities: No clubbing fingers, edema.

Neurological: Minimal weakness and incoordination of muscle movement with loss of associated movements at left arm and leg.

Reflexes: Symmetrical, equal without pathological responses. No definite sensory defects.

生命体征：体温：39.0 ℃，脉搏：110 次/分，呼吸：24 次/分，血压：120/82 mmHg。

患者是一个能言语、意识清晰的老年男性，无急性痛苦面容及发绀。

皮肤：轻度手掌红斑。

头发：无异常。

眼：略突出，眨眼少，余无特殊。

耳鼻喉：除外缺齿，余阴性。

颈部：甲状腺弥漫性增大 2~3 倍，无杂音。

心脏：无增大，无杂音，A2>P2，正常窦性心律。

肺：气管居中，叩诊过清音，呼吸音遥远，双肺下部闻及啰音，无胸膜摩擦音。

腹部：腹膨隆，吸气相肝脏位于右侧肋缘下 3 横指。

脾：未触及。右上腹和上腹部中度压痛。

生殖器：正常。

直肠：前列腺 II 级肿大。

震颤：无杵状指及水肿。

神经系统：左臂和腿部肌肉轻微无力，相关运动丧失，运动不协调。

反射：对称，强度相同，无病理反射，无明确的感觉缺失。

2. 示例 2（Case 2）

Vital signs: T: 37.5, P: 89, irregularly irregular. BP: 139/63, RR: 20, SpO_2 98%.

General: Obese, pale man turning his head side to right side in order to see us. No acute distress.

HEENT: Normocephalic atraumatic. Pupils are equal, round, reactive to light. Discs sharp. Extra ocular muscles intact. Visual acuity/fields as per neuro below. Temporal arteries nontender. Conjunctiva clear.

Neck: No adenopathy. No Jugular vein distension. Carotid pulses 2+ bilaterally.

Pulmonary: Moves air equally bilaterally, though wheezes on auscultation throughout.

Cardiovascular: Irregularly irregular, II / IV systolic crescendo-decrescendo murmur at LUSB, radiating to carotids. No S3, S4. Point of maximum impulse not-displaced.

Abdomen: Obese + normal Bowel sounds. Soft. Nontender. Liver nonpalpable. Liver 8 cm at right midclavicular line by percussion.

Rectal: Brown stool, Occult blood neg in ER.

Pulses: Femoralis R 2+, L +1. Dorsalis Pedis 2+ B. Posterior Tibial 1+ B.

Extremities: No cyanosis, clubbing or edema. Warm, well-perfused.

Neuro: Alert and oriented to person, time, and place; answers questions appropriately.

Cranial Nerves:

I : Able to detect tea at 10 cm.

II : Loss of nasal field R eye, temporal field L eye by confrontation — can detect hand movement in those areas, but can't read vision card at any line. Vision 20/40 B in fields where vision preserved (i.e. if vision card held in front of patients face towards their right).

III, IV, VI: Extraocular movements preserved in all directions.

V : Intact light touch all regions of face; masseter and temporalis muscles 5/5 B.

VII: Muscles of facial expression intact.

VIII: Hearing equal bilateral.

IX, X : Palate symmetric.

XI: Sternocleidomastoid muscle, Trap 5/5.

XII: Tongue midline.

Motor: Strength 5/5: biceps, triceps, quad, plantarflex, dorsiflex. F-N test slight int. Tremor on the left. Rapid alternating movements: symmetric and equal.

Gait: Somewhat unsteady due to visual issues.

Sensory: Intact light touch, pin prick, vibration, proprioception at feet bilateral. Romberg negative.

Reflexes: Biceps, triceps, brachioradialis: 2+B. Patellar, achilles 2+B.

生命体征：体温：37.5 ℃，脉搏：89，绝对不齐，血压：139/63，呼吸：20，血氧饱和度：98%。

一般情况：肥胖，脸色苍白，转头向右，无急性痛苦。

头眼耳鼻喉：头部正常，无创伤。瞳孔等大等圆，对光反射灵敏，视乳头清晰。眼外肌运动正常。视力视野见神经系统检查结果。颞动脉无压痛，结膜干净。

颈部：无淋巴结肿大，无颈静脉怒张。双侧颈动脉搏动 2+。

肺：双侧呼吸动度对称，听诊弥漫性喘息音。

心血管：心律绝对不齐，胸骨左上缘渐增渐减型Ⅱ/Ⅳ级收缩期杂音，向颈部传导，无 S3、S4，最强搏动点无移位。

腹部：肥胖，肠鸣音正常，腹软，无压痛。肝脏未触及。沿右锁骨中线叩诊肝浊音界 8 cm。

直肠：棕色便，急诊隐血阴性。

脉搏：股动脉：右侧 2+，左侧+1；足背动脉：双侧 2+；胫后动脉：双侧 1+。

四肢：无发绀、杵状指或水肿，温暖，灌注良好。

神经系统：神清，人物、时间和地点定向力正常，对答切题。

颅神经：

Ⅰ：10 cm 外可闻及茶味。

Ⅱ：右眼鼻侧视野缺损，左眼颞侧视野缺损（上述区域可感知手部运动，但不能读取视力卡）；双眼其余视野视力20步（视力卡面对患者朝向其右侧）。

Ⅲ、Ⅳ、Ⅵ：各方向眼外肌运动正常。

Ⅴ：面部所有区域触觉正常；双侧咬肌和颞肌肌力 5 级。

Ⅶ：面部表情肌正常。

Ⅷ：双耳听力正常。

Ⅸ、Ⅹ：双腭对称。

Ⅺ：胸锁乳突肌、斜方肌肌力 5 级。

Ⅻ：舌居中。

运动：肌力 5 级：肱二头肌、肱三头肌、股四头肌、跖屈、背屈。指鼻试验大致完整，左侧震颤，快速轮替运动对称且相等。

步态：因视觉问题略有不稳定。

感觉：轻触觉正常，针刺、振动，双侧双足本体感觉正常，Romberg 征阴性；反射：双侧肱二头肌、肱三头肌、桡肌反射 2+，双侧膝反射、跟腱反射 2+。

五、体格检查清单（Checklist）

下面的检查清单可作为体格检查的参考项目。

1. Vital Signs（生命体征）

① Wash hands.

② Ask patient to sit or lie down.

③ General observation.

④ Measure pulse, both radial arteries (rate & rhythm).

⑤ Measure respiratory rate.

⑥ Measure blood pressure (both arms).

⑦ Examine hands, fingers, nails.

洗手。请患者坐或躺下并进行一般性观察。测量双侧桡动脉的脉搏（脉率&节律）、呼吸频率、双臂血压，检查双手手指及指甲。

2. Head and Neck（头颈部）

① Observe face, head, neck & scalp.

② Palpate lymph node, parotid and salivary gland regions.

③ Assess auditory acuity (crude test hearing loss), if hearing loss, perform Weber & Rinne Tests.

Ear: External and internal (otoscope) .

Nose: Observation, nares/mucosa (otoscope) .

Oropharynx:

① Inspect with light from otoscope & tongue depressor → uvula, tonsils, tongue, mucosa.

② "Ahh" to help see back of throat.

③ Inspect teeth & salivary gland ducts.

Thyroid: Observation, palpation.

Eye:

① Observe external eye structures — lid, sclera, pupil.

② Visual acuity (hand-held card — CN Ⅱ) .

③ Visual fields (CN Ⅱ) .

④ Extraocular movements (CN Ⅲ, Ⅳ, Ⅵ) .

Using Ophthalmoscope:

① Examine external eye structures (lids, sclera, pupil, iris, conjunctiva).

② Check pupillary response to light — direct and consensual (CN Ⅱ & Ⅲ).

③ Retinal exam — identifying: optic disc, arteries, veins, color of retina, and macular area.

观察面部、头部、颈部和头皮；触诊淋巴结、腮腺和唾液腺区域；评估听觉敏锐度（粗测），若听力下降，进行 Weber&Rinne 试验。耳：检查外耳&内耳（用检耳镜）；鼻：视诊，鼻孔、黏膜（检耳镜）；咽喉：借助检耳镜及压舌板视诊（悬雍垂、扁桃体、舌、黏膜），发"啊"音帮助查看喉后壁，检查牙齿和唾液腺导管；甲状腺：视诊、触诊。眼：外眼结构（眼睑、巩膜、瞳孔），视力（手持式视力卡——第Ⅱ对颅神经），视野（第Ⅱ对颅神经），眼外肌运动（第Ⅲ、Ⅳ、Ⅵ对颅神经）；检眼镜检查：外眼结构（眼睑、巩膜、瞳孔、虹膜、结膜），瞳孔直接和间接对光反射（第Ⅱ&Ⅲ对颅神经），视网膜检查（视乳头、动脉、静脉、视网膜颜色和黄斑区域）。

3. Pulmonary System（呼吸系统）

Observation & Inspection:

① Generally observe breathing, note if using accessory muscles/general respiratory effort.

② Note shape of chest and spine.

Palpation:

① Assess chest excursion.

② Assess tactile fremitus.

Percussion:

① Percuss posterior lung fields, top to bottom → comparing side to side.

② Identify amount of diaphragmatic descent with inhalation.

③ Percuss right antero-lateral chest (middle lobe) and bilateral chest.

Auscultation:

① Listen with diaphragm to posterior lung fields, top to bottom → comparing left with right.

② Listen to right middle lobe area.

③ Listen to anterior lung fields.

④ Listen over trachea.

视诊：一般性观察呼吸（是否动用辅助呼吸肌），注意胸廓和脊柱的形状；触诊：评估胸壁呼吸动度及语音震颤；叩诊：叩诊后背部（从上到下，双侧对比），评估吸气后横膈肌下降度，叩诊右前外侧胸（右肺中叶）和双侧胸部；听诊：用听诊器膜件听诊后肺野（从上到下，双侧对比），听右肺中叶、前肺野、气管区域等。

4. Cardiovascular System（心血管系统）

① Drape appropriately.

② Examiner stands on right side of patient's body.

③ Patient lying with head of table elevated ~ 30°.

Observation & Palpation:

① Inspect precordium — visible PMI, other contours.

② Palpation of RV and LV (heaves, thrills); Determination of PMI.

Auscultation:

① S1 and S2 in 4 valvular areas with diaphragm; note rate, rhythm.

② Try to identify physiologic splitting S2.

③ Assess for murmurs, characterize if present.

④ Assess for extra heart sounds (S3, S4) with bell over LV.

Carotid Artery:

① Palpation.

② Auscultation.

Internal Jugular Vein:

① Measure jugular venous pressure.

检查者站于患者右侧，患者躺卧位，适当覆盖，检查床头部升高约 30°。视诊&触诊：视诊心前区（最强搏动点及轮廓），触诊左右心室（搏动、震颤），确定最强搏动点；听诊：4 个瓣膜听诊区的 S1 和 S2，注意心率、心律，识别生理性 S2 分裂，评估杂音及其性质，钟形件听诊左室额外心音（S3、S4）；颈动脉：触诊及听诊；颈内静脉：测颈静脉压。

5. Abdomen（腹部）

Lay patient flat. Drape appropriately ─ allowing exposure of abdomen but not rest of body.

Observation & Inspection:

① Shape, scars, color, symmetry, protrusions.

Auscultation:

① Listen with diaphragm to 4 quadrants.

② Note quantity and quality of bowel sounds.

③ Listen for bruits centrally & over renal arteries.

Percussion:

① Percuss all quadrants.

② Percuss liver span.

③ Percuss area of spleen, stomach.

Palpation:

① Palpate all quadrants superficially.

② Palpate all deeply.

③ Try to identify liver edge (with inspiration).

④ Palpate region of spleen.

⑤ Palpate area of aorta.

患者平躺，适当覆盖，充分暴露腹部。视诊：形状，疤痕，颜色，对称性，隆起；听诊：用膜件听诊 4 个象限，注意肠鸣音的数量和质量，腹正中区域及肾动脉杂音；叩诊：叩诊所有象限、肝区、脾区、胃区；触诊：触诊浅表所有象限，深触诊所有象限，肝界（吸气相）、脾区，触诊主动脉区域。

6. Lower Extremities（下肢）

Assess Femoral Area:

① Palpation for nodes.

② Palpate femoral pulse.

③ Auscultation femoral artery (for bruits).

Assess Knees:

① Color, swelling.

② Palpate popliteal artery pulse.

Assess Ankles/Feet:

① Color.

② Temperature.

③ Check cap refill.

④ Check for edema.

⑤ Pulses (dorsalis pedis artery, posterior tibial artery).

评估腹股沟区：触诊淋巴结、腹股沟区搏动，听诊股动脉（杂音）；评估膝盖：颜色、肿胀，触诊腘动脉搏动；评估脚踝/脚：颜色、温度、甲盖充盈、水肿、足背动脉及胫骨后动脉搏动。

7. Neurological System（神经系统）

Higher Cognitive Function:

① Level of consciousness.

② Orientation to time, place, person and situation.

③ Attention — subtract 7 from 100.

④ Memory — 3 objects (dog, number 6 and station) repeat immediately and after 5 minutes.

⑤ Abstract thinking — similarity and difference between orange and ball.

Mental Status Exam:

① Mood — as described by patient.

② Affect — observed by examiner could be congruent or incongruent to described mood.

③ Speech — rate, tone, production.

④ Thought process — linear, goal directed or circumstantial, tangential, disorganized.

⑤ Thought content — delusions, suicidal or homicidal ideations/ intent/plan.

⑥ Insight — good, partial, poor.

⑦ Judgment — what would you do if you found a sealed, addressed, stamped envelope on the ground?

Cranial Nerves:

① CN I — assess smell.

② CN II — visual acuity, visual fields.

③ CN II & III — pupillary response to light.

④ CN III, IV & VI — extra-ocular movements.

⑤ CN V — sensory & motor face; corneal reflex (sensory V, motor VII).

⑥ CN VII — facial expression; smile, puff cheeks, close eyes against resistance.

⑦ CN VIII — hearing assessment, if hearing loss, Webber & Rinne.

⑧ CN IX & X — gag, palate rise.

⑨ CN XI — neck turn/shoulder shrug.

⑩ CN XII — tongue movement.

Motor Testing (Patient Seated):

① Muscle bulk of major groups.

② Tone of major groups.

③ Strength of major groups — shoulders, elbows, wrists, hand, hips, knees, ankle.

Sensory Testing — in distal lower extremities:

① Pain.

② Light touch.

③ Proprioception.

④ Vibration — 128 Hz tuning fork.

Reflexes:

① Biceps.

② Brachioradialis.

③ Triceps.

④ Patellar.

⑤ Achilles.

⑥ Babinski assessment.

Coordination:

① Finger → nose.

② Heel → knee → shin.

③ Rapid alternating finger movements.

Gait, romberg.

Wash hands.

高级认知功能：意识水平，时间、地点、人物和情境定向力，注意力（100 连续减 7），记忆力（检查者说 3 个名词：如猫、数字 6 和车站，让患者立即和 5 分钟后重复），抽象思维（橘子与球的相似性与差异性）。

精神状态检查：情绪（由患者描述），情感（检查者观察到的，可能与所描述的情绪一致或不一致），言语（语速、音调、语量），思维过程（线性的、目标导向或间接的、外围的、无序的），思想内容（妄想、自杀或杀人的想法/意图/计划），洞察力（好、部分、差），判断力（问患者：如果你在地上发现了一个写有地址、贴好邮票、密封的信封，会如何做）。

颅神经：第Ⅰ对：评估嗅觉；第Ⅱ对：评估视力，视野；第Ⅱ&Ⅲ对：瞳孔对光反射；第Ⅲ、Ⅳ、Ⅵ对：眼外肌运动；第Ⅴ对：面部感觉和运动，角膜反射（感觉Ⅴ，运动Ⅶ）；第Ⅶ对：面部表情（微笑，扬起脸颊，对抗阻力闭眼）；第Ⅷ对：评估听力（若听力损失，进行 Weber&Rinne 试验）；第Ⅸ&Ⅹ对：呕吐，抬上腭；第Ⅺ对：转颈、耸肩；第Ⅻ对：舌部运动。

运动检查（患者坐位）：主要肌群肌肉体积、肌力、肌肉强度（肩膀、肘部、手腕、手、臀部、膝盖、脚踝）。

感觉检查（下肢远端）：疼痛觉、触觉、本体觉、振动觉（128 Hz音叉）。

反射：肱二头肌反射、桡反射、肱三头肌反射、膝反射、跟腱反射、巴宾斯基征。

协调：指鼻试验、跟膝胫试验、手指快速轮替运动。

步态，Romberg 征。

洗手。

The practice of medicine is

an art, not a trade;

a calling, not a business;

a calling in which your heart

will be exercised equally

with your head.

— William Osler

进行辅助检查时，医技科室的医师也会说一些祈使句，使患者配合检查，以顺利完成相关检查。

一、句型（Sentences）

(1) After an operation, patients are moved to a recovery area to recuperate.

(2) Breathe in, hold it.

(3) Before an endoscopy, the patient's informed consent must be obtained. Can you give me a sample of your sputum today? If you can't, please bring me a sample on your next visit. I'll give you a sterile glass container to take home with you today.

(4) Can you stand sideways with your right side close to the machine and your arms raised?

(5) Endoscopes can be used to excise disease tissue.

(6) In a moment I'll ask you to take a deep breath in and hold it.

(7) I want you to lie down and just relax.

(8) It's important that you try not to move.

(9) I'm going to go through your questionnaire with you.

(10) It will be over in three quarters of an hour.

(11) It's very important that you put any metal objects into this tray.

(12) I'm going to put some gel on your abdomen. You might find it a bit cold.

(13) I'd like you to lie flat on your back on the table.

(14) I'll move this back and forwards to cover the whole area.

(15) I'm going to give you local anesthesia so that you won't feel any pain.

(16) Keep still.

(17) Now I'm going to take a side view.

(18) Now, let me take a look at the chest X-ray film that you brought with you.

(19) Mr. White, please stir the white, thick fluid in the glass with this spoon and drink it down slowly.

(20) Please stand facing this board.

(21) Put your hands on the back of your hips and your elbows forward. I'll help you.

(22) Push your elbows out.

(23) That's it. All done. I'll just clean you up.

(24) That's it. Fine. You can breathe out now.

(25) Thank you. I'll need to check the film.

(26) The gel is to make sure there's a good contact with your skin.

(27) With an MRI, it's important there are no metallic foreign bodies in the eyes.

(28) We will take your chest X-ray.

(29) Will you please come to the X-ray room? I would like to fluoroscope you.

(30) You don't need any injections.

(31) Your sputum must be examined, then, too.

二、对话示例（Dialogue）

示例 1：验血（Blood Test）

Physician: Ms. Schwarz, from your symptoms it would seem that you have an overactive thyroid gland. We can test this quite simply by doing a blood test to check the level of hormones in your blood.

Physician: Mr. Braun, your father is in a quite poor condition. It seems that he's had diarrhoea for six days and this may have affected his diabetes. As you know, any infection can cause diabetes to get out of control. So we have to check his blood sugar, kidney function and electrolytes level. Because he is already very dehydrated, we'll also give him some fluid. He'll have an X-ray of chest and abdomen. And finally we'll try to find out which particular germ caused his diarrhoea.

示例 2：心电图（ECG）

Physician: Ms. Schwarz, your pulse is a bit irregular. I'm not quite certain why this is but I think we'll have to get a tracing of your heartbeat. I want you to strip down to the waist and also take off your shoes and socks. First of all, this is a completely painless procedure. It's better if you're as relaxed as possible before I start to take the cardiograph. It only takes a few minutes to do the actual test but it takes a bit longer to get you wired up. I'm just putting some cream on your wrists and ankles. Everything is ready. Now just relax as possible as you can.

示例 3：超声检查（Ultrasound Scan）

Physician: Ms. Schwarz, I'd like you to lie down on this table here. This gel helps to get a contact so that the picture is clear. We'll just rub in the gel a little bit and now I'll put on the equipment. Try to keep as still as you can. That's good. Now if you turn your head to the left, you'll be able to see the scan as I'm taking it. As you see, it's just like a television picture. This black part here is the baby's head and this the body. As you can see, it's moving around very well. These dots allow me to measure the baby so we can work out when your baby is due... Everything is finished now.

示例 4：CT 扫描（CT-scan）

Physician: Mr. Braun, I can't find anything wrong with your legs. My bedside evaluation is normal. I expect that you will be alright. However, I think that a CT-scan should be done. This will give you reassurance. The CT-scan is a high-tech kind of an X-ray. It shows important details of your brain. It does not hurt and it is not dangerous. During the examination you will be lying on your back on a stretcher. The technician will advance your head into an arrow tunnel for about 8 minutes. There is nothing to be worried about. There will be enough breathing space around your head. You will be able to speak to the technician by a microphone in the CT-tunnel. The tunnel serves to bring electronic imaging machinery close to your head. Have you ever been afraid of tunnels in your life before?

示例 5：支气管镜检查（Bronchoscopy）

Physician: Mr. Braun, you have to have some investigations done to find out exactly what has caused your problem. Firstly we need to get your chest X-rayed. Then I'd like you to bring a sample of the sputum you coughed up in the morning to the surgery for three times. We'll send them off to the lab for testing to see whether you have got any particular germs. Meanwhile, it's also necessary for you to have a bronchoscopy done. This is an investigation to look down into your lungs through a tube. Therefore we have to admit you into hospital for this investigation. It's not an excessively unpleasant investigation and you'll be given an anaesthetic spray before the tube is passed down into your lungs. Usually it doesn't take more than a few minutes but it may last longer if they need to take samples of the tissue in your lungs, maybe up to 20 minutes. You'll have to take this investigation with an empty stomach, so you shouldn't have any breakfast that day. You'll be able to get home again after the investigation, but you'll have to wait until the anesthetic has worn off before you eat anything.

示例 6：盆腔超声检查（Pelvic Ultrasonography）

Physician: Ms. Schwarz, because of your heavy periods, we must find out if you've become anemic, so I have to take a blood test. I think it will also be necessary for you to have a dilatation and curettage done in hospital. We can probably do this as a day case. It's a very simple procedure and just involves removing a small piece of the lining from inside the womb to find out why our periods have become so heavy. It will also give us a better chance to examine you under the anesthetic. It might also be necessary to do a pelvic ultrasonography. This is a very simple examination which takes a special picture of the lower end of your abdomen to see if the womb is enlarged.

示例 7：平板试验（Treadmill Test）

Physician: Good morning, Mr. Braun. We are going to do a stress test. This is a simple test and will not harm you at all. We need you to walk on this treadmill, which will increase its slope and velocity in a stepwise manner, controlled by me. The nurse here, Sandra, will take your blood pressure every 3 minutes. We will be looking at your ECG recording all the time. Should you feel any chest pain, shortness of breath, dizziness and so on, please let me know. We can stop anytime if needed.

第四节　诊疗方案（Diagnosis and Plan）

疾病的诊断、治疗计划措施以及病情预后等均是患者关注的重要内容，也是医患交流的重点之一，掌握好相关表达有利于实现良好的沟通。

一、诊断（Diagnosis）

1. 句型（Sentences）

(1) Findings on Echocardiogram, along with the ECG and Troponin T suggest...

(2) This is mainly because...

(3) This is why ...

(4) You're suffering from...

(5) You've developed ...

(6) You have...

二、诊疗计划（Plans）

1. 句型（Sentences）

(1) An operation may be advisable.

(2) Can you come again about three days from now?

(3) Can you come again in a few days?

(4) Come again one week later. The results of the X-rays, sedimentation test and examination of your sputum will be available then.

(5) I am putting you on anti-depressants for a short time to help you get back to normal life.

(6) I advise you to go to the university hospital, the sooner the better.

(7) I expect you'll have ....

(8) I'll arrange for you to ....

(9) I'll give you a letter of introduction to the university hospital.

(10) I'm going to start you on medication to ....

(11) I'm going to have you admitted to the coronary care unit.

(12) I'll make you an appointment with ....

(13) I'll refer you to the eye department for examination of your eye grounds.

(14) I think it would be best to enter the hospital immediately, today if possible, and then we can perform more detailed tests.

(15) It can be caused by diet or stress. There are some quite simple tests we can do. If you're still concerned, we can refer you to a hospital.

(16) It's too early to give a definite diagnosis.

(17) There is nothing wrong with you.

(18) This will clear up on its own.

(19) There doesn't seem to be anything wrong with your heart.

(20) They may advise ...

(21) There are a couple of options we could choose. The first option is to try tablets like Prozac that lift you up a bit. The other option is counselling. You'll be given medications to ease the pain and I expect you'll have an angiogram.

(22) This illness is self-limited and will resolve on its own.

(23) We will give you blood transfusion and after your condition improving, we will fluoroscope, and examine the gastric juice and run other tests to confirm the diagnosis.

(24) You should have an operation right now.

三、预后（Prognosis）

1. 句型（Sentences）

(1) Chemotherapy will make you more comfortable.

(2) Could you tell me what we're going to do for you?

(3) Hopefully we can...

(4) His general physician referred him to an oncologist.

(5) He was keen for this to happen.

(6) I'd like to record this consultation so you can listen again if anything isn't clear.

(7) I'd like to see you again next week. Can you come in again next week?

(8) I expect the treatment will improve your pain at least and may get rid of it completely.

(9) I'm afraid your test results aren't very good.

(10) I'm sorry to have to tell you that the news isn't good. Is everything clear to you?

(11) One can never be certain about these things but I'd like to say it's a matter of months rather than years.

(12) There's still a lot we can do to help you.

(13) The patient was disappointed with the news.

(14) The prognosis was discussed with the patient and his wife.

(15) The patient was booked into the ward for further chemotherapy.

(16) The results are consistent with recurrent cancer.

(17) We can never be absolutely certain about the future but you should remain optimistic.

(18) You should remain optimistic.

四、建议（Suggestions）

1. 句型（Sentences）

(1) Carry on drinking lots of fluids.

(2) Cut out fatty foods.

(3) Do you have any questions?

(4) If you aren't feeling better in 7 to 14 days, you really must come back and see me again.

(5) If you keep damaging it, you're going to end up with a long-term problem.

(6) If you feel that things aren't settling, aren't getting back to normal, it's important that you see me again.

(7) If you still have some pain, you can keep taking paracetamol.

(8) Is there anything you'd like to ask?

(9) It's important that you ...

(10) It's very important you don't stop taking the tablets suddenly or your symptoms will return.

(11) I want you to...

(12) Other things might help, like raising the head of your bed. That's one of the simple things we could start you off with. You said you haven't tried indigestion remedies. That's something you could try.

(13) Sometimes off work might help. If you felt that would be helpful, you could take a week off and see how you felt after that. There are a few things about your lifestyle we could address. Perhaps cut down on the amount you're drinking. Giving up smoking would help.

(14) The nurse will give you advice on your diet.

(15) You should try to avoid tight clothing, sitting in deep armchairs and bending, especially after meals.

(16) You should try to give up smoking.

五、对话示例（Dialogue）

示例 1：心绞痛（Angina Pectoris）

Physician: Ms. Schwarz, after having examined you, I'm confident that you're suffering from angina. The heart is a pump. The more you do physically, the harder it has to work. But as we get older, the blood vessels which supply oxygen to the heart begin to harden and get furred up, so they become narrower. They can't supply all the oxygen the heart needs. The result is that pain you fell as angina. Because you're experiencing pain at rest as well as on exertion, I'm going to have you admitted to the coronary care unit right away so that your treatment can start at once. You'll be given drugs to ease the pain and I expect you'll have a coronary angiogram. They may advise surgery or angioplasty — that's a way of opening up the blood vessels to the heart so they can provide more oxygen. You should try to give up smoking. You won't be able to smoke at all in hospital so it's a good time to stop. I expect the treatment will improve your pain at least and may get rid of it completely. We can never be absolutely certain about the future but you should remain optimistic. Do you have any questions?

示例 2：糖尿病（Diabetes Mellitus）

Physician: Mr. Braun, you've suffered from Type 2 diabetes. This is mainly because of significant overweight. Your body isn't producing enough insulin. This is why you feel so thirsty and why you pass urine so frequently. It's also the reason you have this very itchy rash and you have a problem with your eyes. The nurse will give you advice on your diet and I'll arrange for you to a dietitian. I'm going to start you on medication to tablets to control your high blood sugar. You don't need insulin right now but it is possible you might need it in the future. You should try to lose weight and I'll make you an appointment with a podiatrist. It's important for you to take good care of your feet. You should also see your optician every six months for eye checks. Diabetes is a serious condition and can affect your heart, blood pressure, circulation, kidneys and vision but we can limit these problems by controlling your blood sugar. No case of diabetes can be described as mild. I want you to attend the diabetic clinic every two months so we can check your progress. Hopefully we can reduce this to six monthly visits once your condition is under control. Is there anything you'd like to ask?

示例 3：胰腺癌（Pancreatic Cancer）

Physician: Mr. Braun, I'd like to record this consultation so you and Ms. Braun can play back later if anything may not be clear to you today. I am sorry to have to tell you that the scan results aren't very good. It's likely that you've got a recurrence of cancer in your pancreas. That would explain why you've been feeling so tired, and your loss of appetite and weight.

Mr. Braun: Will I need surgery?

Physician: Surgery isn't an option at this stage. Although we can't operate, there is still a lot we can do to help you. You've got tablets for pain relief and we can give you something stronger if you need. We can also start you on a course of chemotherapy to help with your symptoms. This won't cure you but it will make you more comfortable. It's unusual to have any unpleasant side effects with this kind of chemotherapy. I'd like you to see a dietitian for some advice on what to eat and to help get your appetite back.

Mr. Braun: What's my life expectancy? How long have I got?

Physician: One can never be certain about these things. People with this condition vary a great deal. I would be wrong to give you a definite time scale but I'd like to say it's a matter of months rather than years. I am sorry to have to tell you all of this, but my feeling is that it's always best to be honest with people and then you should know what's happening. If you're in agreement, I'd like to book you into Ward 2 to start your chemo. You'll need to come in every week for the next month. Is everything clear to you? (Could you tell me what treatment we're going to give you?) Are there any particular worries you have? I'll be seeing you regularly to keep an eye on things so you can ask me any other questions you may have.

示例 4：高血压（Hypertension）

Ms. Schwarz, you have high blood pressure with headache for 3 years. This condition will not go away by itself. All the necessary tests have been done. They did not show a curable cause of your hypertension. That means you suffer from primary hypertension. But we can treat you with medication. The medicine will bring your blood pressure down to the normal range. It is necessary that you take the medication all the time because its effects expire after about 12 hours. I also recommend a 24-hour ambulatory blood-pressure monitoring. This will allow us to know how is your blood pressure level during the whole day.

示例 5：椎间盘突出（Disc Herniation）

Physician: Well, Mr. White, there's a nerve running behind your knee and your hip and through your spine.

Mr. Braun: Um...

Physician: When you lift your leg, that nerve should slide in and out of your spine quite freely, but with your leg, the nerve won't slide very far. When you lift it, the nerve gets trapped and it's very sore, when I bend your knee, that takes the tension off and eases the pain. If we straighten it, the nerve goes taut and it's painful.

Mr. Braun: Aye.

Physician: Now what is trapping the nerve? Well, your MRI scan confirms that you've got a damaged disc in the lower part of your back.

Mr. Braun: Oh, I see.

Physician: The disc is a little pad of gristle which lies between the bones in your spine. Now, if you lift heavy loads in the wrong way, you can damage it. And that's what's happened to you. You've damaged a disc. It's pressing on a nerve in your spine so that it can't slide freely and that's the cause of these pains you've been having.

Mr. Braun: Uhuh.

Physician: Now we're going to try to solve the problem first of all with a maximum of twenty four hours' bed rest and with strong painkillers so that you'll be able to get moving again as soon as possible. Bed rest for too long can make things worse. We'll also give you some physio to ease your leg and back. I can't promise this will be entirely successful and we may have to consider an operation at a later date.

示例 6：十二指肠溃疡（Duodenal Ulcer）

Physician: Mr. Braun, your stomach has been producing too much acid. This has inflamed an area in your bowel. It's possible that your stressful job has aggravated the situation. This is quite a common condition and there is an effective treatment. It doesn't involve surgery.

示例 7：痴呆（Dementia）

Physician: Ms. Schwarz, your mother is in the early stage of dementia which is a condition of the brain in older people which causes loss of memory, particularly recent memory. Sometimes people with dementia also have delusions. Her personality may change, for example she may become rude or aggressive. Her mood may become very up and down. At this stage she can stay at home with some help but her condition will deteriorate and she will need to go into care in the long term.

示例 8：甲状腺功能低下（Hypothyroidism）

Physician: Mr. Braun, the cause of your problem is your thyroid gland which is situated here in your neck. The hormones from this gland affect all areas of your body. If the gland isn't working properly, many things can go wrong. For example, it can cause weight gain and hair loss. This is a common condition and the treatment is simple.

示例 9：先天性心脏病（Congenital Heart Disease）

Physician: Mr. Braun, your baby has a heart condition which developed when she was growing in the womb. Some babies with this condition are born looking blue but it's also possible for the blueness to develop after a few weeks. The blood flow in the heart becomes abnormal and this causes your baby to grunt and have difficulty in feeding. Fortunately, there is an operation for treatment of this condition. It's extremely likely to bring your baby into a normal life.

As to diseases, make a habit of two things

— to help, or at least, to do no harm.

— Hippocrates

用药是临床医疗活动中非常重要的环节，药物名称、剂型、剂量、服药方法的准确交代，不良反应的监测对患者病情恢复至关重要。而医患交流沟通的效果直接决定患者服药的依从性，甚至疗效，因此临床医师应该高度重视此类沟通。

一、词汇（Vocabulary）

Antiemetics: to stop or prevent vomiting

Anthelminthics: to eliminate worms

Anti-inflammatory drugs: to decrease inflammation

Antitussives: to stop coughing

Bronchodilators: to reduce bronchial spasms

Diuretics: to help the patient to produce urine

Mucolytics: to liquefy viscid bronchial mucus

Sedatives/tranquilizers: to induce tranquility or sleep

Spasmolytics: to relax smooth muscles and relieve cramps

Analgesics: to relieve pain

Antibiotics: to eliminate infections

Antacids: to neutralize acid in the stomach

Antipyretics: to bring the temperature down

Antihypertensives: to bring the blood pressure down

Emetics: to help the patient to vomit

Antiasthmatics: to treat bronchial asthma

Vasodilators: to dilate blood vessels and improve circulation

药物剂型: Capsules, injection, ointment, paste, pessary, powder, solution, spray, suppository, syrup, tablets, inhaler

不良反应: Allergy, abdominal discomfort, gastric problems, dizziness, nausea, vomiting, diarrhea, respiratory problems, shortness of breath, breathlessness, high blood pressure, renal failure, kidney disorders, visual disturbance, palpitations.

常用缩写：p.c. = after food, q.d.s = four times a day, s.c. = subcutaneous, s.l. = sublingual, p.o = by mouth, c.c. = with meals, p.r.n = as required, i.v. = intravenous, infus = fusion

ACEI: Benazepril, Captopril, Enalapril, Fosinopril, Lisinopril

ARB: Candesartan, Eprosartan, Irbesartan, Losartan, Telmisartan, Valsartan

Benzodiazepines: Alprazolam, clonazepam, diazepam, flurazepam, lorazepam, oxazepam

Beta blockers: Atenolol, bisoprolol, esmolol, metoprolol, carvedilol, labetalol, sotalol

Calcium channel blockers: Amlodipine, diltiazem, felodipine, nicardipine, nimodipine, verapamil

Cephalosporin

Cefadroxil, cefazolin, cephalexin, cephradine

Cefaclor, cefamandole, cefotetan, cefprozil, cefuroxime

Cefdinir, cefditoren, cefixime, cefoperazone, cefotaxime, cefpodoxime, ceftazidime, ceftizoxime, ceftriaxome

Cefepime

Fluoroquinolones

Ciprofloxacin, gatifloxacin, levofloxacin, lomefloxacin, moxifloxacin, norfloxacin, sparfloxacin

HMG-CoA reducteas inhibitors

Atorvastatin, fluvastatin, lovastatin, pravastatin, simvastatin

二、常用动词搭配（Verbs）

apply + cream, liniment, ointment, spray, tincture

chew + lozenge, pill, tablet

inhale from + spray, inhaler, nebulizer

massage in + cream, liniment, ointment, spray, tincture

put on + cream, liniment, ointment, spray, tincture

rub in/on + cream, liniment, ointment, spray, tincture

swallow + capsule, lozenge, pill, tablet

take + capsule, lozenge, pill, tablet

use + cream, liniment, ointment, spray, tincture

三、句型（Sentences）

(1) Apply some talcum powder to your skin.

(2) Apply a thin coat of the ointment every evening and then cover with a wet dressing.

(3) Dip a cotton bud in this tincture and apply to your gums.

(4) Drop some mixture on a sugar cube. Shake the mixture well before taking.

(5) Insert one of these suppositories into the vagina before going to bed.

(6) Pour an ampoule of this solution into boiling water and inhale it for five minutes.

(7) Mix 15 drops in a cup of water and gargle 2-3 times a day.

(8) Place this pill under your tongue and allow it to dissolve. If you are unable to swallow this tablet, break it in half or crush it into a power.

(9) Rub a thin layer of this cream on your skin.

(10) Swallow this tablet without chewing.

(11) Take this tablet half an hour before meals.

(12) Take a pinch of this powder and mix it with some water.

(13) This is a bitter tablet, so take it with some sort of juice.

(14) Take this capsule with some water.

(15) Use three drops of these eye drops every evening.

四、对话示例（dialogue）

示例 1

Physician: You seem to have localized skin rash caused by a bacterial infection. This means that you will have to take some antibiotics. Are you allergic to any medicine?

Mr. Braun: Yes, actually, I had quite a bad reaction once when I took penicillin. I felt a choking sensation and my tongue was badly swollen.

Physician: Ok, then I'll prescribe an antibiotic without penicillin. You'll have to take one tablet three times a day, preferably immediately after eating.

Mr. Braun: Is there some kind of lotion that I could use on my skin?

Physician: Yes, I can also prescribe an anti-inflammatory ointment or some talcum powder. Both should help reduce the burning and itching sensation. I recommend the ointment, but I'll prescribe whichever you prefer. Which would you rather like to use?

Mr. Braun: Then I'll take the ointment, as you suggested.

Physician: You should apply it whenever you need to. Do you feel that you need some painkillers?

Mr. Braun: Yes, that would be quite helpful, I haven't been able to do anything since this started; it hurts so badly.

Physician: Well, that should clear it up. If everything looks good you won't have to come back again. However, if the symptoms don't go away after a week, make sure you come back and see me again.

示例 2

Mr. Braun: Doctor, you prescribed some tablets for my pneumonia. By the evening my face was flushed and itching, and I had come out in a rash.

Physician: Oh, I'm afraid you must be allergic to that medicine, I'll prescribe something else that shouldn't affect you.

Mr. Braun: I came down with the flu so I took the aspirin you suggested; however, by the next morning I had an upset stomach. I'm afraid to continue with it, but I'm still running a fever.

Physician: Aspirin sometimes affects the stomach. I think you should take Paracetamol instead, it doesn't cause stomach problems.

Mr. Braun: I've been feeling dizzy since I started taking the new blood pressure tablet. When I bend down, I'm afraid I'll fall over.

Physician: Your pressure has come down a little low and that's causing the dizziness, so we'll adjust the dosage of your tablet.

Mr. Braun: I've been feeling sick since I started taking this new medicine. I've had an upset stomach since then.

Physician: Oh, I'm sorry. We have to change the tablets to stop the nausea.

示例 3

Physician: Mr. Braun, you have a stent implanted in your left anterior descending artery. As you know, it is a drug-eluting stent, and to avoid thrombotic complications you need to take a combined antiplatelet regime for at least 6 months. Clopidogrel, 75 mg one pill daily at breakfast time, along with ASA 100 mg, one pill daily at breakfast time. Besides, we need to control your blood pressure, so we'll continue on enalapril 5 mg and bisoprolol 2.5 mg, as before the admission. Remember that bisoprolol has some secondary effects that you have already noticed (fatigue and sexual dysfunction). Should you have any other problems, please contact me as soon as you can. Here you have your complete written prescription with my phone number at the bottom.

第六节 知情同意（Informed Consent）

治疗措施的知情同意过程，一般需要交代患者的病情及诊断，拟采取治疗措施的目的、过程、风险和获益，其他替代治疗措施的风险和获益，以及不接受拟定治疗措施的风险等。

一、句型（Sentences）

(1) Mr. Braun, this is the informed consent sheet. Take your time to read it carefully. I can answer all your questions and clear your doubts. Would you mind please sign this form, if you don't have any questions?

(2) Informed consent was obtained from the patient after discussing risks and benefits of the procedure.

二、对话示例（Dialogue）

Physician: Mr. Braun, Good morning. I hope I didn't wake you up.

Mr. Braun: Good morning, Doctor. What news do you have for me?

Physician: Well, Mr. Braun, we have been discussing your case in our morning meeting. We have got all results of your tests. Unfortunately, we find that there is a "growth" in your colon, and it doesn't seem to be good. The reason why you have felt so tired lately is because you are slowly losing blood through your stools, and that is why you required a blood transfusion recently.

Mr. Braun: But is it "bad," Doctor?

Physician: Well, as I have told you, it doesn't seem to be good. However, we are lucky that we caught it relatively early and it has not gone very far. Therefore, we recommend you have it removed. If we do the operation now, the chances of it spreading to other parts of your body will be minimal.

Mr. Braun: Is it a serious operation, Doctor?

Physician: In your case, we can remove the tumor by open, standard surgery, or via laparoscopic surgery. There are no other real treatment options. Lap surgery makes the operation longer but the scars will be minimized, normally offering a faster recovery. However, unfortunately, in both cases we will have to do a "colostomy". It means that, for a period of time you will have to wear a plastic bag on your belly to receive your stools. If everything goes well, we will reconnect your colon a few months later, so that you will be able to go to the toilet normally.

Mr. Braun: Yes, I have heard about that.

Physician: This is a "big" operation, and there are some risks that you should know. First, there are possibilities of bleeding, infection, wound opening, and heart problems after the operation. However, you are still a young man and quite fit, so, these perioperative risks are relatively low.

Mr. Braun: When will the second operation take place?

Physician: Once we have confirmed that your liver is clean and that the tumor is gone during follow up, we will talk about this operation with you, but you should know that it may take months to years. This situation will affect your quality of life. However, it is the best solution we can offer to cure your disease or at least keep you tumor free as long as possible.

Mr. Braun: When will the operation be?

Physician: If you agree with the procedure, we could schedule it for next Wednesday. After the operation, you normally spend about two weeks in the hospital to get you used to the new situation.

Mr. Braun: OK, I guess I have no other choice.

Physician: I think it is your best option. This is a written form that explains all the details about the procedure and the possible risks and benefits. I will leave it here for you and your family. Read it carefully and please sign it when you have no questions on the operation and then give it to your nurse. Thank you. See you later, Mr.Braun.

Mr. Braun: Thank you. See you tomorrow, Doctor.

第七节　手术（Operation）

　　手术（操作）中不可避免地会与患者、同事进行必要的沟通以便手术/操作顺利进行。一般情况下，此过程中的沟通都言简意赅。手术（操作）前、后也因相关事宜与患者或亲属沟通，此时的沟通则较为细致全面。

一、术中与患者（In Operation）

　　(1) Breathe in deeply.

　　(2) Breathe out deeply and hold your breath.

　　(3) Don't breathe, don't move.

　　(4) Let me know if this hurts (to check the local anesthetic is working properly).

　　(5) Keep still.

　　(6) Push as if you were going to have a bowel movement (Valsalva maneuver).

　　(7) Take a deep breath and hold your breath.

　　(8) This can sting (when you are injecting the anesthetic).

　　(9) You may feel some palpitations now. It is normal. Do not worry.

　　(10) You may feel some chest pain. It's nothing to worry about.

　　(11) You will feel a burning sensation in your head and stomach during injection of contrast material. It is also normal.

二、术前与亲属（Before Operation）

　　Physician: Mr. Braun, your father/husband/mother/wife/son/daughter is about to undergo a coronary angiogram. Depending on findings, it will take approximately 30-60 minutes. The procedure does not need a general anesthetic, only local anesthesia, so your father will remain conscious. I will let you know how the procedure went as soon as we finish.

三、术后交代（After Operation）

Physician: Mr. Braun, I am afraid your father's condition is critical. He will be transferred to the ICU. Unfortunately, we have not been able to cross the stenosis so the patient will be transferred to the department of cardiovascular surgery where he will receive an operation. There has been a serious complication. Your father is being transferred to the operating room where he will be operated on. We (the surgeon and I) will inform you of the situation as soon as the operation is finished.

第八节 查房（Visit/Ward Round）

查房是日常医疗活动中的重要内容，涉及医生患者间以及医生间、医护间的对话，对话的重点多围绕患者的病情及诊治安排等。

1. 句型（Sentences）

(1) Are you feeling alright / well?

(2) Are your bowels acting properly?

(3) Are your bowels regular?

(4) Can we get an ultrasound and blood cultures and make a decision tomorrow?

(5) Can we get some more fluids going in and try sips of water later today as long as there's no further vomiting.

(6) Do you have any appetite? Do you have difficulty breathing?

(7) Have you ever had this experience before?

(8) How long has this been going on?

(9) How long have you had this trouble?

(10) How are you feeling now?

(11) How's your sleep?

(12) Is the cut still painful?

(13) I'm still having a lot of pain, is that normal?

(14) I've changed Miss Brown's antibiotics and she's apyrexial now.

(15) I think we need to change the antibiotics and do another X-ray in 48 hours.

(16) I'd like to see what happens over the next 24 hours and have another look in the morning.

(17) Mr. Braun had a chest X-ray yesterday — it shows a decrease in consolidation of the left lung.

(18) Mr. Braun is working really hard on his exercises.

(19) Mrs. Rose is three days post-op — she's feeling so much better.

(20) Ms. Schwarz is doing really well on the stairs.

(21) What did you eat yesterday?

(22) What seems to be bothering you?

(23) What's the matter with you?

(24) When do you think I'll be able to go home, doctor?

(25) Will I need another operation, doctor?

(26) Will I be able to walk properly soon, doctor?

(27) We had a bit of a rough day yesterday but things seem to be much more settled now.

(28) We seem to have shifted some of the consolidation.

(29) We'll take you to the theatre tomorrow and try to sort all this out, is that alright with you Miss Rose?

(30) You're almost ready to go home now — isn't that right Mrs. Schwarz?

2. 对话示例（Dialogue）

Physician: Good morning, Mr. Braun.

Mr. Braun: Good morning.

Physician: How do you feel today? Did you sleep well?

Mr. Braun: I think I am doing quite OK. The wound is a bit sore and tonight I could not sleep very much.

Nurse: He had a peak of temperature at about 2:00 am, but it resolved with 1 gram of acetaminophen and it has not recurred.

Physician: OK. Let me listen to your chest with a stethoscope. Have you had any cough?

Mr. Braun: No, not really.

Physician: The urinary catheter is still in, we will take it out now. (To the nurse): Please send a urine sample to the laboratory to look for white cells. The wound looks quite nice. The operation was only a couple of days ago and it is normal to be a bit uncomfortable.

Mr. Braun: Thank you.

Physician: Thank you. Take it easy, we will order an X-ray and a blood test, but everything seems to be OK. See you tomorrow.

Nurse: Shall we review the treatment?

Physician: Of course. Please leave an order to take a blood culture if the temperature rises again. We will also take the central line out, but leave the peripheral catheter in situ until we have the results of the white cell count. Let's check the treatment.

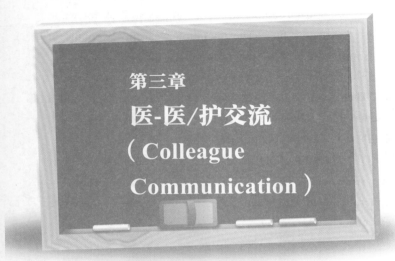

第三章
医-医/护交流
（Colleague
Communication）

Medicine is learned by the bedside
and not in the classroom.
Let not your conceptions of disease
come from the words heard in the lecture room
or read from the book.
See and then reason and compare and control.
But see first.

— William Osler

病例汇报可以出现于临床医疗过程中的各个场景，如查房、疑难病例讨论等。需注意的是，病例汇报应该简洁明了、重点突出。此类口语汇报中常使用短句和短语，以提高效率。

新患者的病史汇报应该围绕此次就诊的主要问题进行汇报，内容包括主诉、现病史（重要症状及伴随症状）、既往史、用药史、个人史、阳性/阴性体征以及重要检查的阳性结果，初步诊断、鉴别诊断及诊疗计划等。老患者则可省略之前已汇报的基础情况，着重汇报患者疾病及不适的变化情况、治疗的反应、新症状和新的异常发现以及进一步的诊疗计划。

一、完整的病例汇报（Completed Presentation）

（一）内容（Contents）

1. Introduction（Chief Complaint）

I'd like to present Mr. Braun, a 34-year-old farmer.

2. History of Present Illness

who presented with a one-month history of breathlessness,

who was electively admitted for evaluation of exertional dyspnea,

who comes into clinic for follow-up of...

3. Related Symptoms

He also complained of ankle swelling which he'd had for two weeks.

4. Past Medical History

His other medical problems include insulin-requiring diabetes for 12 years, complicated by retinopathy, polyneuropathy, and nephropathy.

He has a long history of chronic obstructive lung disease with steroid dependence and the requirement for home oxygen therapy.

There was no relevant past history (He underwent appendectomy).

5. Social History

He was married with one son. He smoked 30 cigarettes a day and drank about 60 ml of alcohol per week.

6. Family History

His father died of myocardial infarction at the age of 42. His mother was alive and well.

7. Findings on Examination

On examination, he was obese...

On auscultation, there were coarse crepitations at the right base.

示例 1

On physical examination, the temperature was 37.4 °C, the pulse 84 beats per minute, the blood pressure 140/63mmHg, the respiratory rate 18 breaths per minute, and the oxygen saturation 92% while he was breathing ambient air. The weight was 61 kg, the height 158 cm, and the body-mass index 24.7. The patient did not appear ill. The abdomen was nondistended, with normal bowel sounds and no tenderness on palpation. The spleen was palpable. Multiple right inguinal lymph nodes were enlarged, measuring 2 to 5 cm in maximal diameter; the nodes were hard, nonmobile, and mildly tender, and there were no overlying skin changes. Multiple left inguinal lymph nodes measured 1 to 2 cm in maximal diameter. There was no lymphadenopathy in the occipital, posterior auricular, anterior cervical, posterior cervical, axillary, epitrochlear, or supraclavicular region. There were no rashes or skin lesions. The remainder of the physical examination was normal.

体格检查显示：体温 37.4 °C，脉搏 84 次/分，血压 140/63 mmHg，

呼吸 18 次/分，血氧饱和度 92%。体重 61 kg，身高 158 cm，体重指数 24.7。患者无明显病容，腹部无膨隆，肠鸣音正常，触诊无压痛。脾脏可触及。右侧腹股沟多个淋巴结肿大，最大直径为 2～5 cm，质硬、不活动，轻度压痛，表皮无明显变化。左侧腹股沟多个淋巴结，最大直径为 1～2 cm。枕部、耳后、颈前、颈后、腋窝、滑车上或锁骨上区淋巴结未见肿大。全身无皮疹或皮损。其余检查正常。

示例 2

On examination, the temperature was 37.6 °C, the pulse 66 beats per minute, the blood pressure 132/82 mmHg, the respiratory rate 16 breaths per minute, and the oxygen saturation 97% while the patient was breathing ambient air. The weight was 76.2 kg; the last recorded weight, which had been obtained 4 years earlier, was 81.8 kg. The patient did not appear to be ill but was in mild distress because of abdominal pain. Erythematous, follicular papules and hyperpigmented nodules, some with central erosion and ulceration, were distributed on the trunk, arms, legs, face, and scalp. Examination of the heart and lungs was normal. Bowel sounds were present, and the abdomen was soft, with tenderness on palpation of the right upper quadrant, but was not distended. There was right axillary lymphadenopathy but no submandibular, cervical, supraclavicular, or inguinal lymphadenopathy.

体格检查显示：体温 37.6 °C，脉搏 66 次/分，血压 132/82 mmHg，呼吸 16 次/分，血氧饱和度 97%。体重 76.2 kg；4 年前末次记录的体重 81.8 kg。患者似乎未患病，但因腹痛而处于轻微痛苦中。躯干、手臂、大腿、面部和头皮上分布有红斑、滤泡性丘疹和色素沉积结节，部分伴有中央糜烂和溃疡。心肺检查均正常。肠鸣音存在，腹部柔软，右上象限触痛，无腹部膨隆。右侧腋窝淋巴结肿大，下颌下、颈部、锁骨上或腹股沟淋巴结无肿大。

8. Investigation Results

We did a chest X-ray which showed...

9. Diagnosis and Differential Diagnosis

The possible diagnosis is ...

示例 1：An Undiagnosed Problem

The most likely reason for Ms. Schwarz's rash is eczema. Her skin dryness and pruritus, and her family history of atopy are all consistent with eczema, as is the history of worsening in the winter and after frequent swimming. She also has a classic distribution on the hands and elbow creases. A less likely possibility is scabies, which frequently affects the hands. However, Ms. Schwarz's skin between the wrists and elbows is spared, which would be atypical for scabies.

示例 1：未确诊的问题

施瓦茨女士皮疹最可能的原因是湿疹。她皮肤干燥伴瘙痒，冬季和频繁游泳后病情恶化，这一特异性家族史均与湿疹相一致。她的皮疹也经典性分布于手和肘部皱褶。一个较低的可能性是疥疮，它经常影响到双手。然而，施瓦茨女士的手腕和肘部间的皮肤未受累，这对疥疮而言是不典型的。

示例 2：An Exacerbation of a Chronic Problem

The most likely reason for Mr. Braun's CHF exacerbation is medication non-adherence due to both costs and confusion. He reports filling his medications less often than monthly because even the co-pay is expensive, which is confirmed by his pharmacy. Although he manages his own medications, he is unable to accurately describe what each is for, or his dosing schedule. A second possibility is a new ischemia event; however, he's had no chest pain or tightness, and initial ECG and cardiac enzymes were negative. Finally, a upper respiratory infection could have precipitated this exacerbation, as he had low grade fever, cough, and rhinorrhea last week. However, those symptoms have resolved as his edema and shortness of breath have progressed, making this possibility less likely.

示例 2：慢性问题的恶化

布劳恩先生慢性心力衰竭恶化最可能的原因是费用和糊涂导致的药物不依从。他说即便共同付费，药费也很昂贵，其服药的次数少于每月应服次数。尽管自己管理药物，他却无法准确描述每种药物的用途或给药计划。第二种可能性是新发缺血事件。但他没有胸痛或紧箍感，最初的心电图和心肌酶均阴性。最后，上呼吸道感染可能导致了此次恶化，因其上周有低烧、咳嗽和流涕，但随着他的水肿和呼吸困难的进展，上述症状已消失，所以这种可能性比较低。

示例 3：Routine Follow-up of a Chronic Problem

Mr. Braun's type 2 diabetes is well controlled, with most recent HbA1c of 6.8. He reports excellent adherence to diet and exercise, as well as metformin and dapagliflozin. He has no evidence of retinopathy or neuropathy on exam and urine for microalbumin was negative.

示例 3：慢性问题常规随访

布劳恩先生的 2 型糖尿病控制良好，最近的糖化血红蛋白为 6.8。他报告了良好的饮食、运动以及二甲双胍和达格列净依从性。检查中没有发现视网膜病变或神经病变的证据，尿微量白蛋白呈阴性。

10. Plan & Treatment

Treatment:

Aspirin was administered.

Antibiotic was employed.

Antihistamine and aminophylline were prescribed to him.

We gave him intravenous furosemide and ...

11. Outcome

He responded to treatment and was discharged home with...

（二）病例示例（Cases）

1. 新患者（New Patients）

Chief Complaint:

Mr. Braun is a 55-year-old male with AIDS, on HAART, with preserved CD4 count and undetectable viral load, who presents for the evaluation of fever, chills and a cough over the past 7 days.

主诉：布劳恩先生是一名 55 岁艾滋病男性患者，接受高活性抗反转录病毒治疗，CD4 数保留，病毒载量未检测到，因 7 天前出现发烧、寒战和咳嗽而就诊。

History of Present Illness:

Mr. Braun has been known to be HIV + since 2005. Until one week ago, he had been quite active, walking up to two miles a day without feeling short of breath. Approximately 1 week ago, he began to feel dyspneic with moderate activity. Three days ago, he began to develop subjective fevers and chills along with a cough productive of red-green sputum. One day ago, he was breathless after walking up a single flight of stairs and spent most of the last 24 hours in bed.

现病史：2005 年被确诊 HIV 感染。直至 1 周前他一直很活跃，日行 2 英里（3.2 km）而无呼吸困难。约 1 周前中等强度运动使他出现呼吸困难。自述 3 天前出现发热、寒战，伴咳红绿色痰。1 天前上一层楼即感呼吸困难，就诊前 24 小时大部分时间都在床上。

Past HIV History:

Diagnosed with HIV in 2005, done as a screening test when found to have gonococcal urethritis.

Was not treated with HAART at that time due to concomitant alcohol abuse and non-adherence.

Diagnosed and treated for PJP pneumonia 2008.

Became sober in 2010, at which time interested in HAART. Started on Atripla, a combination pill of Efavirenz, Tenofovir, and Emtricitabine. He's taken it ever since, with no adverse effects or issues with adherence. CD4 count three months ago was 800 and viral load was undetectable.

He has no history of asthma, COPD or chronic cardiac or pulmonary condition. No known liver disease. Hepatitis B and C are negative.

既往 HIV 病史：2005 年因淋球菌性尿道炎筛查诊断 HIV 感染，当时因酗酒和依从性差，未接受 HAART 治疗。2008 年诊断肺孢子虫肺炎并治疗。2010 年戒酒接受 HAART 治疗，服用依非韦伦、依诺福韦和恩曲他滨联合治疗。此后他坚持服药，无不良反应或依从性问题。3 个月前 CD4 数为 800，病毒载量无法检测到。无哮喘、慢性阻塞性肺病或慢性心肺疾病史。无已知的肝病史。乙肝和丙肝阴性。

System Review:

Negative for headache, photophobia, stiff neck, focal weakness, chest pain, abdominal pain, diarrhea, nausea, vomiting, urinary symptoms, leg swelling, or other complaints.

系统回顾：无头痛、畏光、颈部僵硬、局灶性无力、胸痛、腹痛、腹泻、恶心、呕吐、泌尿系统症状、腿肿或其他症状。

Other Past Medical History:

Hypertension eight years, no other known vascular disease. GERD, Gonorrhea as above, Alcohol abuse above and now sober — no known liver disease. No relevant surgeries.

其他既往史/社会史：高血压史 8 年，无其他已知的血管疾病史。曾患胃食管返流疾病、淋病，酗酒已戒，无已知肝病史，无手术史。

Medications and Allergies:

Atripla, 1 po qd, Omeprazole 20 mg, 1 po, qd, Valsartan 150 mg, 1 po, qd, Naprosyn 250 mg, 1-2 po, bid, prn.

No allergies.

药物及过敏史：

依非韦伦、恩曲他滨、依诺福韦，每次 1 片，每日 1 次；奥美拉唑 20 mg，每次 1 片，每日 1 次；缬沙坦 150 mg，每次 1 片，每日 1 次；萘普辛 250 mg，每次 1 ~ 2 片，每日 2 次，按需使用。无过敏史。

Family History:

Both of the patient's parents are alive and well (his mother is 76 and father 81). He has one brother, 42 yr old, who is also healthy. There is no family history of heart disease or cancer.

家族史：父母都健在（母 76 岁，父 81 岁）。一个兄弟，42 岁，体健。无心脏病或癌症家族史。

Social History:

Patient works as an engineer for a large firm. He lives alone in an apartment in the city. Smokes one pack of cigarettes per day for 18 years. No current alcohol use. Denies any drug use. Has sex exclusively with men, last partner six months ago.

社会史：一家大公司当工程师。独居公寓。吸烟 18 年，每天 1 包。目前不饮酒，未吸毒，只与男性发生性关系，6 月前曾有伴侣。

Physical Examination:

Seated on a gurney in the ER, breathing through a face-mask oxygen delivery system. Breathing was labored and accessory muscles were in use. Able to speak in brief sentences, limited by shortness of breath. Vital signs: Temp 39.2 ℃, Pulse 92, BP 148/90, Respiratory Rate 25, O_2 Sat (on 40% Face Mask) 95%. HEENT: No thrush, No adenopathy. Lungs: Crackles and Bronchial breath sounds noted at right base. No wheezing or other abnormal sounds noted over any other area of the lung. Dullness to percussion was also appreciated at the right base. Cardiac: JVP less than 5 cm; Rhythm was regular. Normal S1 and S2. No murmurs or extra heart sounds noted. Abdomen and Genital exams: normal. Extremities: No clubbing, cyanosis or edema; distal pulses 2+ and equal bilaterally. Skin:

no eruptions noted. Neurological exam: normal.

体格检查：坐于急诊室轮床上，面罩吸氧，呼吸用力，动用辅助呼吸肌。可说简短句子，因呼吸困难受限。生命体征：体温 39.2 ℃，脉搏 92，血压 148/90，呼吸 25，氧饱和度（面罩吸氧浓度 40%）95%。头眼耳鼻喉：无鹅口疮，无淋巴结肿大。肺：右肺底部湿啰音和支气管呼吸音。其他区域无喘息或其他异常呼吸音。右肺底叩诊浊音。心脏：颈静脉压力小于 5 cm，节律规整。S1 和 S2 正常。无杂音或额外心音。腹部和生殖器检查：正常。四肢：无杵状指、发绀或水肿；远端脉搏 2+，双侧对等。皮肤：无破损。神经系统检查：正常

Labs and Imaging:

WBC: 15*10^9/L, Neutrophils ratio: 82%;

Normal liver and renal function.

Room air blood gas: pH of 7.45/ pO$_2$ of 56/pCO$_2$ of 32.

Sputum gram stain remarkable for an abundance of polys along with gram positive diplococci.

CXR is remarkable for dense right lower lobe infiltrates without effusion.

实验室影像学检查：

白细胞：15×10^9/L，中性粒细胞比值：82%；肝肾功能正常。血气分析：pH 7.45，pO$_2$ 56，pCO$_2$ 32。痰革兰氏染色：大量花粉和革兰氏阳性双球菌。胸片：右下叶致密浸润影，无积液。

Diagnosis and Plan:

① Acute community acquired pneumonia:

Mr. Braun is an HIV+ male with preserved CD4 count and undetectable viral load while on HAART, who presents with an acute pulmonary process. The rapid progression, focality of findings on lung exam and chest x-ray, along with the sputum gram stain suggest a bacterial infection, in particular Streptococcal Pneumonia. Other pathogens to consider include influenza, H Flu and Legionella. His presentation, compliance with Pneumocystis pneumonia prophylaxis, reasonably intact immune system and statement that his current illness seems different then past Pneumocystis pneumonia infection would argue against this as the etiologic agent. Mycobacterial infection also seems unlikely. Viral infections and neoplastic processes like CMV or Kaposi's Sarcoma of the lung do not typically give this clinical presentation nor should they occur given his level of immune function. In addition, he received a flu vaccine two months ago. The data does not support the existence of either a primary cardiac or noninfectious pulmonary process.

诊断和计划：

① 急性社区获得性肺炎：

布劳恩先生是一名 HIV+男性，接受 HAART 治疗，CD4 数保留，病毒载量无法检测到，表现为急性肺部疾病病程。进展快、肺部检查和胸部 X 光检查结果及痰革兰氏染色提示有细菌感染，尤其是链球菌性肺炎。其他需要考虑的病原体包括流感、H 型流感和军团菌。他的临床表现、预防肺孢子虫肺炎的依从性、完整的免疫系统，及目前疾病表现与既往患过的肺孢子虫肺炎感染不同，因而肺孢子虫不应是此次患病的致病源。分枝杆菌感染可能性也较低。病毒感染和肿瘤，如巨细胞病毒或肺卡波西氏肉瘤，通常不会出现这种临床表现，也不会在他这样的免疫功能水平发生。此外，2 个月前他还接种了流感疫苗。这些数据也不支持原发性心脏疾病或非感染性肺部疾病的存在。

The current plan for his pneumonia is as follows:

(i) Continue Ceftriaxone and Azithromycin started in the ED for acute CAP.

(ii) Follow up on cultures of sputum and blood; will try to narrow coverage based on final cultures.

(iii) Obtain rapid flu test.

(iv) Continue Atripla.

(v) Continue O_2, with goal to keep sats greater than 92%.

(vi) IV fluid replacement with Normal Saline at 125 ml/h for next 24 hours to correct mild hypovolemia, with plan to reassess volume status at that time.

(vii) If patient does not show improvement (or worsening) and cultures are unrevealing, consider bronchoscopy as a means of making more definitive diagnosis.

(viii) Monitored care unit, with vigilance for clinical deterioration.

目前肺炎治疗计划如下：

继续使用于急诊室启用的头孢曲松和阿奇霉素治疗急性社区获得性肺炎。复查痰培养和血培养，尝试根据最终培养结果缩小抗菌药物覆盖范围。进行快速流感检测。继续服用 Atripla。继续吸氧，血氧饱和度目标大于 95%。静脉补液纠正轻度低血容量，生理盐水替代，125 mL/h，持续 24 h，复评容量状态。如果病情无改善或恶化，而培养物也是阴性，则考虑进行支气管镜检查，进一步明确诊断。监护病房，警惕临床恶化。

② Hypertension:

Given significant pneumonia and unclear clinical direction, will hold Valsartan. If BP > 160 and or if clear not developing sepsis, will consider restarting.

② 高血压：

鉴于严重的肺炎和临床走向不明，暂停缬沙坦。若血压>160 和/或明确不出现脓毒症，将考虑重新启动。

③ DVT Prophylaxis:

Immobile and ill, which makes him high risk; Low molecular weight heparin.

③ 深静脉血栓预防：

制动及生病使其深静脉血栓风险增高，使用低分子量肝素。

2. 老患者（Known Patients）

Daily Presentations（日常汇报）

Introduction:

This is Mr. Smith, a 66-year-old man, Hospital Day 2, being treated for right leg cellulitis.

介绍：史密斯先生，65 岁，住院第二天，因右腿蜂窝织炎接受治疗。

Events of the Past 24 hours:

MRI of the leg, negative for osteomyelitis.

Evaluation by Orthopedics, who I&D'd (incision&drainage) a superficial abscess in the calf, draining a moderate amount of pus.

24 小时内病程：

腿部 MRI 检查：无骨髓炎；骨科会诊：切开引流小腿浅表脓肿，引流适量脓液。

PE Remarkable for:

Patient appears well, states leg is feeling better, less painful. T max 38.6 ℃ yesterday, T Current 36.5 ℃; Pulse range 62-84; BP 130-166 s/72-80 d; O_2 sat 99% Room Air. Ins/Outs: 3.5 L in (2 L NS, 1.5 L po)/Out 4 L urine. Right lower extremity redness now limited to calf, well within inked lines — improved compared with yesterday; bandage removed from the I&D site, and base had small amount of purulence; No evidence of fluctuance or undrained infection.

体格检查：

患者状况良好，自述腿部感觉更好，疼痛减轻；昨日最高体温 38.6 ℃，目前 36.5 ℃；脉搏 62 ~ 84；血压：收缩压 130 ~ 166，舒张压 72 ~ 80；室内血氧饱和度 99%。出入量：入 3.5 L（2 L 生理盐水，饮入 1.5 L），出 4 L 尿液。右下肢发红，现仅限于小腿，在墨水线内，与昨日相比有所改善；绷带已从切开引流处拆除，伤口基底部有少量的脓液；无波动感或未引流感染。

Labs and Imaging Remarkable for:

Creatinine 72.1, down from 130.5 yesterday. WBC $8.2*10^9$/L, down from $13*10^9$/L. Blood cultures from admission still negative. Gram stain of pus from yesterday's I&D: + PMNS; Culture pending. MRI lower extremity as noted above — negative for osteomyelitis.

实验室和影像学检查：

肌酐 72.1，昨日 130.5。白细胞 8.2×10^9/L，之前 13×10^9/L。入院时的血培养结果仍为阴性。昨日切开引流液的革兰氏染色：多形核粒细胞+，待培养结果。下肢 MRI：骨髓炎阴性。

Diagnosis and Plan:

This is a 66-year-old man, hospital day 2, being treated for lower extremity cellulitis and abscess.

① Cellulitis complicated by abscess, which has now been adequately drained. Exam improved and felt better. Likely organism is Staph, covering for MRSA until cultures back. Continue Vancomycin for today. Ortho to reassess I&D site, though looks good. Follow-up on cultures: if MRSA, will transition to PO Doxycycline; if MSSA, will use PO Dicloxacillin.

诊断和计划：这是一名 66 岁的男性，住院第二天，正在治疗下肢蜂窝织炎和脓肿。

① 蜂窝织炎伴脓肿，现已充分引流，病灶改善，患者感觉良好。致病菌很可能是葡萄球菌，抗感染覆盖耐甲氧西林金黄色葡萄球菌，直至培养结果回来。今天继续使用万古霉素。尽管切开引流伤口看起来不错，再请骨科会诊。追踪培养结果：如果是耐甲氧西林金黄色葡萄球菌，则口服多西环素；如果是甲氧西林敏感金黄色葡萄球菌，则口服双氯西林。

② Hypertension:

When admitted, outpatient anti-hypertensive medications held as blood pressure was low due to sepsis. Now BP is climbing back to hypertensive range. No symptoms. Given AKI, will continue to hold ACE-inhibitor; will likely wait until outpatient follow-up to restart. Add back amlodipine 5 mg/d today.

② 高血压：

入院时暂停降压药，因脓毒症导致血压较低。现在血压上升超正常范围，无症状。鉴于急性肾损伤，将继续暂停 ACEI，可能待到门诊随访后重新启动，今日恢复氨氯地平 5 mg/d。

③ Renal:

Now back to baseline kidney function, which is normal. On admission AKI due to sepsis. All improved as expected with control of infection.

③ 肾：

现在肾功能恢复至正常。入院时因脓毒症引起急性肾损伤。随着感染的控制均如预期改善。

④ Disposition:

Anticipate d/c tomorrow on po antibiotics (pending final culture results as above to determine best oral med). Wound care teaching with nurse today (wife capable and willing to assist, she'll be in this afternoon). Set up follow-up to reassess wound and cellulitis within 1 week.

④ 安排：

预计明日出院，带口服抗生素（据最终培养结果以确定最佳口服药物）。护士今日教伤口护理（妻子有能力且愿意协助，今天下午到场）。预约随访，1 周内重新评估伤口和蜂窝织炎。

二、简略的病例汇报（Brief Presentation）

（一）病例示例（Cases）

示例 1

Mr. Collins is a 66-year-old security guard. He presented with a six week history of pain in the legs. The pain, which was located around the ankles, has been increasing in intensity and was associated with local tenderness. On routine questioning, he said that he had had a morning cough with small amounts of white sputum for many years. He produced, once, some steaks of blood in the sputum. There was no relevant previous medical history. He smokes 20 cigarettes per day and drinks 15-20 gram of alcohol everyday. On examination, there was marked tenderness around the lower legs above the ankles and knees. There were crackles at the left base posteriorly in the chest. There was nothing else abnormal to find on examination except for clubbing of the fingers. Chest X-ray showed consolidation in the left lower lobe. Bronchoscopy and biopsy showed adenocarcinoma of the lung and computed tomography scan showed that this was not resectable. Treatment with chemotherapy has resulted in temporary improvement in the chest X-ray but the leg pain has continued to prove difficult to control.

柯林斯先生是一名 66 岁的保安。他有 6 周的腿部疼痛病史，疼痛位于脚踝周围，强度不断增加，并与局部压痛有关。在例行询问中，他说他多年来早上咳嗽伴少量白痰。曾有一次出现痰中带血块。既往无相关病史。他每天抽 20 支烟、饮 15～20 g 酒精。体格检查发现脚踝和膝盖以上的小腿周围有明显的压痛。左后背基底部闻及啰音。除外杵状指，余无异常发现。胸片显示左下肺叶实变。支气管镜检查和活检提示肺腺癌，计算机断层扫描显示这是不能被切除的。化疗使胸片检查结果得以暂时改善，但腿部疼痛仍难以控制。

示例 2

I'd like to present Mr. White who's a 60-year-old taxi driver who presented to the Outpatient Clinic with a three-month history of increasing shortness of breath and ankle swelling. He had a chronic cough with purulent sputum and occasional hemoptysis. Of note in his past medical history was that he's had a partial gastrectomy in 2000. On examination, he was pale. He was apyrexial. He had leg oedema, but no clubbing or lymphadenopathy. And examination of his chest was entirely normal. His liver was palpable five centimeters below the costal margin, and was smooth and non-tender, and there was also a scar from his previous operation.

我介绍一下怀特先生，60 岁的出租车司机，因呼吸困难和脚踝水肿 3 月到门诊就诊。他有慢性咳嗽伴脓性痰，偶尔咯血。值得注意的既往病史是他在 2000 年接受了部分胃切除术。体格检查发现他脸色苍白，无发热，腿部水肿，无杵状指或淋巴结肿大。胸部检查完全正常。肝脏肋缘下 5 cm 可触及，光滑，无压痛，还有既往手术疤痕。

示例 3

This 30-year-old female employee presented for the treatment of recurrent headaches. Her headaches are primarily in the suboccipital region, bilaterally but worse on the right. Sometimes there is radiation toward the right temple. She describes the pain as having an intensity of up to 5 out of 10, accompanied by a feeling of tension in the back of the head. When the pain is particularly bad, she feels that her vision is blurred. This problem began to develop three years ago when she commenced work as a data entry clerk. Her headaches have increased in frequency in the past year, now occurring three to four days per week. The pain seems to be worse toward the end of the work day and is aggravated by stress. Aspirin provides some relief. She has not sought any other treatment. Otherwise the patient reports that she is in good health. There is no family history of headaches. Examination revealed an otherwise fit-looking young woman with slight anterior carriage of the head. Cervical active ranges of motion were full and painless except for some slight restriction of left lateral bending and rotation of the head to the left. These motions were accompanied by discomfort in the right side of the neck. Cervical compression of the neck in the neutral position did not create discomfort. However, compression of the neck in right rotation and extension produced some right suboccipital pain. Cranial nerve examination was normal. Upper limb motor, sensory, and reflex functions were normal. With the patient in the supine position, static palpation revealed tender trigger points bilaterally in the cervical musculature and right trapezius. Motion palpation revealed restrictions of right and left rotation in the upper cervical spine, and restriction of left lateral bending in the mid to lower cervical spine. Blood pressure was 110/70. Holding the neck in extension and rotation for thirty seconds did not produce dizziness. There were no carotid bruits. The patient was diagnosed with cervicogenic headache due to chronic postural strain. The patient undertook a course of treatment consisting of cervical and upper thoracic spinal manipulation three times per week for two weeks. Manipulation was accompanied by trigger point therapy to the paraspinal muscles and stretching of the upper trapezius. Additionally, advice was provided concerning maintenance of proper posture at work. The patient was also instructed in the use of a cervical pillow. Furthermore, the intensity of her headaches declined throughout the course of treatment. Based on the patient's reported progress during the first two weeks of care, she received additional two treatments in each of the subsequent two weeks. During the last week of care, she experienced no headaches and reported feeling generally more energetic than before commencing care. Following a total of four weeks of care (10 treatments), she was discharged.

30 岁的女性雇员来院治疗复发性头痛，头痛主要位于双侧枕下区域，右侧更严重，有时放射至右侧太阳穴，疼痛强度高达 5 分，并伴后脑勺的紧箍感。头痛特别严重时，她会觉得自己视力模糊。她 3 年前开始做数据录入员时症状开始出现。在过去 1 年里，她的头痛频率增加，现在每周发作 3~4 d。头痛似乎在工作日结束时更严重并可因压力而加重，阿司匹林可缓解部分疼痛，她还没有寻求过任何其他的治疗。此外，该患者说她健康状况良好，没有头痛家族史。体格检查：一个健康的年轻女性，头部轻微的前倾。除头部向左侧弯曲及头部向左旋转轻微受限，颈椎活动范围正常且无痛。这些动作伴随右侧颈部不适。正中体位压迫颈部不会造成不适。但在头部右旋右展位时压迫颈部会导致右枕下疼痛。颅神经检查正常。上肢运动、感觉和反射功能正常。患者仰卧位静态触诊发现，双侧颈部肌肉组织和右侧斜方肌触发点压痛。运动触诊发现上颈椎左右旋转受限，中下颈椎左侧弯曲受限。血压 110/70。保持颈部过伸旋转位 30 s 不会导致头晕。未闻及颈动脉杂音。患者因慢性姿势性紧张而被诊断为颈源性头痛。患者接受了一个疗程的治疗，包括颈椎和上胸椎推拿，每周 3 次，连续 2 周。推拿治疗联合椎旁肌肉的触发点治疗和上斜方肌的伸展。此外还给予了工作中保持正确姿势、使用颈枕的建议。她的头痛强度在整个治疗过程中逐步下降。根据治疗前 2 周的情况，她在随后 2 周内接受 2 种额外的治疗。在治疗的最后 1 周，她没有头痛且感觉比治疗前更精力充沛，经总计 4 周的治疗（10 次治疗）后出院。

示例 4

Mrs. Schwarz is an 88-year-old lady who was admitted from her nursing home this morning. She has a background of COPD and heart failure; she has oxygen at the nursing home and is normally hoisted between bed and chair. She presents with a 3-day history of cough, productive of green sputum, worsening shortness of breath and reduced oral intake. Her GP started her on amoxicillin and 30 mg prednisolone yesterday. Mrs. Schwarz normally takes inhalers and antihypertensives as listed here. On examination, she is requiring 35% oxygen to maintain saturations of 90%; she is tachypneic at a rate of 24 bpm and is using her accessory muscles of respiration. Her temperature on admission was 38.4 °C. Auscultation of the chest reveals bibasal crepitations, worse on the left, and global expiratory wheeze. There is an associated increase in vocal resonance on the left side of the chest. There is significant dependent oedema evident bilaterally up to the knees. The chest X-ray shows cardiomegaly, blunting of both costophrenic angles and left lower zone consolidation. Her arterial blood gas on 35% O₂ showed a partially compensated respiratory acidosis with a pH of 7.34, pO₂ of 64, pCO₂ of 53 and a base excess of - 4. In summary, this 88-year-old lady presents pyrexial with a productive cough on a background of COPD and heart failure with X-ray changes consistent with a left lower lobe pneumonia. My leading differential diagnosis is pneumonia causing by infective exacerbation of COPD; I have sent bloods for analysis, including blood cultures, and I have started antibiotics, steroids, nebulizers and fluids as per the hospital guidelines.

88 岁的施瓦茨夫人今天早上从养老院入院。她有慢性阻塞性肺病和心力衰竭病史；她在养老院吸氧，通常活动限于床和椅子间。她咳嗽 3天，咳绿色痰，呼吸困难加重、食欲下降。她的全科医生昨日开始给予她口服阿莫西林和 30 mg 泼尼松龙。施瓦茨夫人日常使用如下所列的吸入制剂和抗高血压药物。体格检查发现她需要吸入浓度 35% 的氧气以达90% 的氧饱和度，她呼吸急促，24 次/分，动用辅助呼吸肌。入院体温为38.4 °C。胸部听诊发现双肺基底噼啪声，左侧更重，及弥漫性呼气喘息。左胸语音共振也相应增强。双下肢至膝盖处均有明显水肿。胸片显示心脏扩大，双侧肋膈角变钝，左下肺实变。给予 35% 氧气吸入时动脉血气显示部分代偿性呼吸性酸中毒，pH 7.34，pO₂ 为 64，pCO₂ 为 53，剩余碱 - 4。总之，这位以慢性阻塞性肺病和心力衰竭为基础病的 88 岁女性，发热、咳嗽等症状及 X 片改变，符合左下叶肺炎诊断。主要鉴别诊断是由慢性阻塞性肺病感染性加重所致的肺炎，已送血检，包括血培养，已根据医院指南启动抗感染、激素、雾化和液体治疗。

在日常与同事的交流沟通中，辅助检查结果的描述、讨论也是诊疗活动中重要的内容。

一、句型（Sentences）

An ultrasound scan of the liver revealed (demonstrated, showed) reduction of metastases.

二、描述范例（Examples）

1. 验血（Blood Tests）

示例

Dr. Lewis: Blood levels of electrolytes, glucose, and lactate dehydrogenase were normal, as were the results of renal function and liver function tests. Tests for antibodies to hepatitis B virus (HBV) surface antigen and antibodies to HBV core antigen were positive. The N-terminal pro-B-type natriuretic peptide level was 4850 pg per milliliter, the d-dimer level 2487 ng per milliliter, and the lactate dehydrogenase level 458 U per liter.

2. 心电图（ECG）

示例 1

Dr. Lewis: The very abnormal ECG revealed a rate of approximately 33/min, a single long pause of approximately 4 seconds between ventricular complexes with atria activity, widened QRS complexes in keeping with (R)BBB. Deep T wave inversion in Ⅱ, Ⅲ, AVF and some chest leads V4-V6. Deep QRS complexes in V2 and V5 in keeping with

LVH. One atrial ectopic. QT interval is normal.

示例 2

Dr. Lewis: the repeated ECG showed normal sinus rhythm, frequency 75 bpm, electrical axis at 75. normal PR interval (0.13s), abnormal QRS duration (0.19s) with morphology of right bundle branch block and T-wave inversion in right precordial leads and premature ventricular ectopic beat.

示例 3

Dr. Das: Good morning Dr. Lewis. Would you please help me with this ECG?

Dr. Lewis: Of course Dr. Das. Let's see ... It is a sinus rhythm tracing with a normal axis; I don't see any conduction abnormalities, but it seems to me that the ST-segment is a little bit elevated. What are the patient's symptoms?

Dr. Das: He complains of typical chest pain.

Dr. Lewis: When did the pain start?

Dr. Das: A few days ago. He has a fever and cough.

Dr. Lewis: Well, Dr. Lewis. I think we have made a diagnosis. It is not an acute coronary syndrome because the ST-changes are widespread through all precordial and limb leads. Otherwise, according to patient symptoms it seems to me that your patient could have pericarditis. Let's perform an ultrasound scan.

3. 超声检查（Ultrasound Scan）

示例 1

Dr. Lewis: Bedside ultrasonographic examination of the heart revealed a hyperdynamic left ventricle.

示例 2

Dr. Lewis: Abdominal ultrasonography revealed an ill-defined mass (9.0 cm by 5.6 cm) in the right lobe of the liver, with no evidence of dilatation of intrahepatic bile ducts.

4. 胸片（CXR）

示例

Dr. Lewis: A portable chest radiograph showed persistent asymmetric lung opacities. Also seen were new septal lines, increased thickening of the right minor fissure, and increased perihilar haziness.

5. CT

示例 1

Dr. Lewis: Computed tomography of the chest, performed after the administration of intravenous contrast material, revealed multiple prominent cardiophrenic lymph nodes ($\leqslant 1$ cm in maximal short-axis diameter) predominantly on the right side. There were also multiple enlarged axillary lymph nodes ($\leqslant 3.4$ cm in maximal short-axis diameter) on the right side, including some with central necrosis.

示例 2

Dr. Lewis: CT of the abdomen and pelvis revealed multiple ill-defined hypodensities throughout the right lobe and in the fourth segment of the liver, with the largest measuring 2.7 cm by 2.0 cm. Trace perihepatic ascites and mild splenomegaly were present, with the spleen measuring 13.5 cm in craniocaudal dimension.

6. 核磁共振（MRI）

示例

Dr. Lewis: Magnetic resonance imaging of the liver, performed after the administration of intravenous contrast material, revealed multiple areas of abnormality in the right lobe that corresponded to the lesions seen on CT, with the largest measuring 3.1 cm by 6.3 cm by 3.5 cm. The lesions had mild peripheral hyperintensity on T2-weighted images and restricted diffusion on diffusion-weighted images. On images obtained during the portal venous phase, the lesions had peripheral enhancement with central hypoenhancement. On images obtained 4 minutes after the administration of contrast material, the lesions had a "cluster of grapes" appearance. Mild splenomegaly was also detected.

第三节 手术操作（Operation）

手术操作的成功完成需要医生间、医护间的紧密配合，而围绕手术的工作交流则非常重要。

一、句型（Sentences）

(1) A phone call? Tell him I'll call back later; I can't break scrub now.

(2) Can I have a facemask?

(3) Could you give me a hood?

(4) Can I have this image magnified, please?

(5) Could you please collimate the image to minimize my hand exposure?

(6) Can you let me know where the shoe covers are?

(7) Can I have a 0.014 guidewire?

(8) Can I have a hydrophilic guidewire?

(9) Can I have a 5F introducer?

(10) Can I have a 16-ga needle?

(11) Can I have a torque device?

(12) Can I have a stiffer guidewire, please?

(13) Do we have lead aprons?

(14) Give me the ventricular lead please.

(15) Give Dr. Lewis a pair of shoe covers (thyroid shield, lead apron).

(16) Give me a JL4 please.

(17) Give me a 3X20 balloon please.

(18) I'll need a pair of lead gloves.

(19) I'm going to double-glove for this case.

(20) I'll take 8 under and 8½ on top.

(21) I left my radiation badge in my locker.

(22) I'd rather use a Swan-Ganz catheter.

(23) I can now see the stent. I'll use an Amplatz goose neck snare.

(24) I'll go scrub in a minute.

(25) Is the patient monitored yet?

(26) Let's connect the generator. Double-check the electric threshold.

(27) May I have my gown tied?

(28) May I have another pair of gloves, please?

(29) May I have a pair of lead gloves?

(30) My scrubs top is soaked. I need to change it.

(31) Mary, I forgot my thyroid shield. Could you put one on me?

(32) This lead apron is too small. Can I have a larger one?

(33) There is a blood strain on my scrub pants (trousers).

(34) Tie me up, please.

(35) What size gloves do you take? 8.

(36) Would you tie my gown?

(37) Where are the lead aprons?

(38) We've had an iliac dissection. Page the vascular surgeon.

值班也是医疗活动中重要的环节，涉及与同事们就医疗活动的各种交流。

一、句型（Sentences）

(1) Admitted for chest pain.

(2) Admitted for oncologic work up.

(3) Can the patient be repositioned in the left lateral decubitus position?

(4) Diagnosed with ...

(5) Everybody was either pre-call or post-call.

(6) From then on, it's "only" every third night for the rest of the month. My pager is not working properly. May I have some fresh batteries?

(7) Her pager number is 888999.

(8) I am returning a page. How can I help you?

(9) I am on again tonight.

(10) I am scheduled to be on with ...

(11) I concur with the previous report.

(12) I get the weekend off. I've just reviewed your patient's ECG, and wanted to discuss the findings with you.

(13) I got only one hit.

(14) Is Mr. Braun having neurological symptoms?

(15) I would like to obtain more information on her presentation and past.

(16) It is not emergent.

(17) I'll contact the technologist.

(18) I'll follow up on these studies.

(19) I'll be post-call on Tuesday and Friday.

(20) I'm the cardiologist on call.

(21) In the ICU on Day 10.

(22) In your next golden weekend...

(23) I want to inform you about the findings.

(24) Is the patient under contact precautions?

(25) Is the patient intubated?

(26) It seems like every walk-in needs a brain CT.

(27) I've woken up from my pre-call sleep.

(28) I will get some extra help to move the patient.

(29) I will set up the ultrasound machine.

(30) Patient's medical record number 123456.

(31) Post-call days.

(32) Resident coming on call.

(33) Resident finishing call.

(34) Thank you for contacting me regarding Mr. Braun's CT.

(35) There are two studies pending.

(36) The contact person for the patient is Dr. Lewis.

(37) That makes me suspicious of ...

(38) The IV (line) has fallen out.

(39) The next study of choice would be ...

(40) The nurse has called for the patient.

(41) Transport is on the way.

(42) To order a coronary CT, ...

(43) To obtain it as a "next available" study, ...

(44) To page the referring physician, ...

(45) We must replace the IV line.

(46) Who is on call today?

二、对话示例（Dialogue）

示例 1

Dr. Lewis: This is Dr. Lewis. I am the cardiologist on call. I am returning a page. How can I help you?

Nurse: Dr. Lewis, you didn't return a page from the vascular surgeon?

Dr. Lewis: I haven't been paged in the last couple of hours.

Nurse: Is your pager working properly?

Dr. Lewis: I'm afraid it's not working properly. Do you have some fresh batteries?

示例 2

ER physician: Hello, I would like to order a brain MRI and CT of the abdomen and pelvis for Ms. Schwarz. She was recently diagnosed with lung cancer and is being admitted for abdominal pain and further oncologic workup.

Radiologist: Is Ms. Schwarz having neurologic symptoms or is the brain MRI for staging?

ER physician: For staging.

Radiologist: If the patient is having no neurologic symptoms and the brain MRI is requested for staging only, it is reasonable to obtain it as a "next available" study, since it is not emergent. The CT of this abdomen and pelvis is appropriate, given the patient's symptoms and will be done emergent. I will contact with the CT technologist.

示例 3

Cell phone rings.

Surgeon: This is Dr. Lewis speaking.

ER Physician: Is that vascular surgery?

Surgeon: Yes, what do you have for me?

ER Physician: I'm calling you about a 55-year-old man, smoker, who came to the ER about 20 minutes ago. He reported acute abdominal pain that started some 4 hours ago. He collapsed because of the pain, though he has recovered by himself. I'm calling you because we have just got the lab results and his hemoglobin is down to 7. I think he might have a ruptured abdominal aneurysm.

Surgeon: Has he had a CT? Did you palpate a pulsatile abdominal mass?

ER Physician: Not yet, I have just ordered it. I think it would be finished in about 30 minutes. I did not really palpate anything because the patient is quite obese.

Surgeon: OK, it looks like a possibility. Listen, I will get the OR ready. Please call me once the patient is at the CT unit and we will transfer him immediately. Meanwhile, ask for six packs of red blood cells and try to keep his blood pressure under control, especially with fluids.

ER Physician: Sure.

Surgeon (new call): May I speak to the anesthesiologist on duty, please?

Operator: Just a second.

Surgeon: Would you call the cardiovascular nurses as well? Please tell them to get OR number 9 ready, we have an emergent operation — a ruptured aneurysm.

Operator: OK, Dr. Lewis. Here is the anesthesiologist.

Anesthesiologist: Yes, Dr. Lewis? What's up?

Surgeon: Who is this?

Anesthesiologist: This is Dr. Holmes speaking.

Surgeon: Good evening, Dr. Holmes. We seem to have a ruptured aneurysm in a 55-year-old patient. The patient is on his way to the CT and I would like to transfer him directly to the OR. At the moment, his BP is still holding.

Anesthesiologist: We have just finished an operation, no problem. I will send someone to OR 9. Give me a call once the CT is finished and we'll escort the patient to the OR.

Surgeon: Thanks, Dr. Holmes. See you in a while.

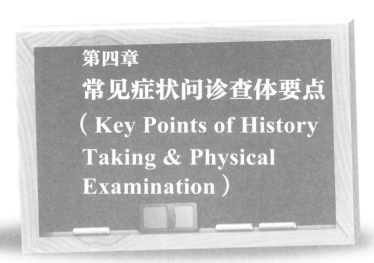

第四章
常见症状问诊查体要点
（Key Points of History Taking & Physical Examination）

To study the phenomena of disease without books
is to sail an uncharted sea,
while to study books without patients
is not to go to sea at all.
— *William Osler*

以常见的症状为线，掌握与其相关的病史采集、体格检查及鉴别诊断中常用的医学专业英语词汇，是学习、掌握医学英语的重要基础。本章总结介绍临床常见症状问诊、查体、鉴别、诊断中常用医学专业词汇。

一、发热（Fever）

1. Chief Complaint

The patient is a 50-year-old male with hypertension who complains of fever for one week.

2. History of the Present Illness

Degree of fever, time of onset, pattern of fever; shaking chills (rigors), cough, sputum, sore throat, headache, neck stiffness, dysuria, urinary frequency, back pain; night sweats; vaginal discharge, myalgias, nausea, vomiting, diarrhea, anorexia. Chest or abdominal pain; ear, bone or joint pain; recent acetaminophen use. Exposure to tuberculosis or hepatitis; travel history, animal exposure; recent dental, GI procedures; Foley catheter; antibiotic use, alcohol, allergies.

3. Past Medical History

Cirrhosis, diabetes, heart murmur, recent surgery; AIDS risk factors.

4. Medications

Antibiotics, acetaminophen.

5. Social History

Alcoholism.

6. Physical Examination

General Appearance: Note whether the patient appears, septic, ill, or well. Toxic appearance, altered level of consciousness, dyspnea, diaphoresis.

一、发　热

1. 主　诉

50 岁高血压男性患者，发热 1 周。

2. 现病史

发热程度，起病时间，发烧方式；颤抖，咳嗽，痰，喉咙痛，头痛，颈项强直，排尿困难，尿频，背痛；盗汗；阴道分泌物，肌痛，恶心，呕吐，腹泻，厌食。胸腹部痛；耳，骨或关节痛；近期对乙酰氨基酚用药史。结核病或肝炎接触史；旅游史，动物接触史；近期口腔、消化道手术史；留置尿管；使用抗生素，酒精，过敏。

3. 既往史

肝硬化，糖尿病，心脏杂音，近期手术史；艾滋病相关危险因素。

4. 药物史

抗生素，对乙酰氨基酚。

5. 社会史

酗酒。

6. 体格检查

一般情况：注意对患者的一般印象，如脓毒症、病中或状况良好。中毒表现，意识水平变化，呼吸困难，发汗。

Vital Signs: Temperature (fever curve), respiratory rate (tachypnea), pulse (tachycardia), BP.

Skin: Pallor, delayed capillary refill; rash, purpura, petechia (septic emboli, meningococcemia). Pustules, cellulitis, abscesses.

HEENT(Head, Eyes, Ears, Nose, Throat): Papilledema, periodontitis, tympanic membrane inflammation, sinus tenderness; pharyngeal erythema, lymphadenectasis, neck rigidity.

Breast: Tenderness, masses.

Chest: Rhonchi, crackles, dullness to percussion (pneumonia).

Heart: Murmurs (endocarditis), friction rub (pericarditis).

Abdomen: Masses, tenderness, hepatomegaly, splenomegaly; Murphy's sign (right upper quadrant tenderness and arrest of inspiration, cholecystitis); shifting dullness, ascites. Costovertebral angle tenderness, suprapubic tenderness.

Extremities: Cellulitis, infected decubitus ulcers or wounds; IV catheter tenderness (phlebitis), calf tenderness, Homan's sign; joint or bone tenderness (septic arthritis). Osler's nodes, Janeway's lesions (peripheral lesions of endocarditis).

Rectal: Prostate tenderness; rectal mass, fissures, and anal ulcers.

Pelvic/Genitourinary: Cervical discharge, cervical motion tenderness; adnexal or uterine tenderness, adnexal masses; genital herpes lesions.

Neurologic: Altered mental status.

7. Labs

CBC, blood Culture, glucose, BUN, creatinine, UA, urine Gram stain, Culture; lumbar puncture; skin lesion cultures, bilirubin, transaminases; tuberculin skin test; Chest X-ray; abdominal X-rays; CT scans.

生命体征：体温（热型），呼吸频率（呼吸急促），脉搏（心动过速），血压。

皮肤：苍白，毛细血管充盈延迟；皮疹，紫癜，瘀点（脓毒血症性栓子，脑膜炎球菌血症）。脓疱，蜂窝织炎，脓肿。

头眼耳鼻喉：视乳头水肿，牙周炎，鼓膜炎，鼻窦压痛；咽部红斑，淋巴结肿大，颈部僵硬。

乳房：压痛，包块。

胸部：干啰音，湿啰音，叩诊浊音（肺炎）。

心脏：杂音（心内膜炎），心包摩擦音（心包炎）。

腹部：包块，压痛，肝大，脾大；墨菲氏征（右上腹压痛和吸气受阻，胆囊炎）；移动性浊音，腹水。肋脊角压痛，耻骨上区压痛。

肢体：蜂窝织炎，褥疮感染或伤口；静脉导管压痛（静脉炎），小腿压痛，Homan 征；关节或骨骼压痛（脓毒性关节炎），Osler 结节，Janeway 损害（心内膜炎的外周病灶）。

直肠：前列腺压痛；直肠肿块，直肠裂和肛门溃疡。

骨盆/泌尿生殖系统：宫颈分泌物，宫颈运动痛；附件或子宫压痛，附件包块；生殖器疱疹病变。

神经系统疾病：精神状态改变。

7. 实验室检查

血常规，血培养，血糖，血尿素氮，肌酐，尿酸，尿液革兰氏染色，血、尿培养；腰穿，皮肤病变培养，胆红素，转氨酶；结核菌素皮肤试验；胸腹部 X 片；CT 等。

8. Differential Diagnosis

Infectious Causes: Abscesses, mycobacterial infections (tuberculosis), cystitis, pyelonephritis, endocarditis, wound infection, diverticulitis, cholangitis, osteomyelitis, IV catheter phlebitis, sinusitis, otitis media, upper respiratory infection, pharyngitis, pelvic infection, cellulitis, hepatitis, infected decubitus ulcer, peritonitis, abdominal abscess, perirectal abscess, mastitis; viral infections, parasitic infections. Malignancies: Lymphomas, leukemia, solid tumors, carcinomas. Connective Tissue Diseases: Lupus, rheumatic fever, rheumatoid arthritis, temporal arteritis, sarcoidosis, polymyalgia rheumatica.

Other Causes: Atelectasis, drug fever, pulmonary embolism, pericarditis, pancreatitis, factitious fever, alcohol withdrawal. Deep vein thrombosis, myocardial infarction, gout, porphyria, thyroid storm.

Medications Associated Fever: Barbiturates, isoniazid, nitrofurantoin, penicillin, phenytoin, procainamide, sulfonamides.

8. 鉴别诊断

感染性原因：脓肿，分枝杆菌感染（结核），膀胱炎，肾盂肾炎，心内膜炎，伤口感染，憩室炎，胆管炎，骨髓炎，静脉导管静脉炎，鼻窦炎，中耳炎，上呼吸道感染，咽炎，盆腔感染，蜂窝组织炎，肝炎，褥疮创口感染，腹膜炎，腹腔脓肿，直肠周围脓肿，乳腺炎；病毒感染，寄生虫感染。恶性肿瘤：淋巴瘤，白血病，实体瘤，癌。结缔组织疾病：狼疮，风湿热，类风湿关节炎，颞动脉炎，结节病，风湿性多肌痛。

其他原因：肺不张，药物热，肺栓塞，心包炎，胰腺炎，人为发热，戒酒。深静脉血栓形成，心肌梗死，痛风，卟啉症，甲状腺危象。

药物热：巴比妥类药物，异烟肼，硝基呋喃妥因，青霉素，苯妥英钠，普鲁卡因酰胺，磺胺类药物。

二、头痛（Headache）

1. Chief Complaint

The patient is a 55-year-old female complaining of headache for 4 hours.

2. History of the Present Illness

Quality of pain (dull, band-like, sharp, throbbing), location (retro-orbital, temporal, suboccipital, bilateral or unilateral), time course of typical headache episode; onset (gradual or sudden); exacerbating or relieving factors; time of day, effect of supine position. Age at onset of headaches; change in severity, frequency; awakening from sleep; analgesic or codeine use; family history of migraine. "The worst headache ever" (subarachnoid hemorrhage).

Aura or Prodrome

Visual scotomata, blurred vision; nausea, vomiting, sensory disturbances.

Associated Symptoms

Weakness, diplopia, photophobia, fever, nasal discharge (sinusitis); neck stiffness (meningitis); eye pain or redness (glaucoma); ataxia, dysarthria, transient blindness. Lacrimation, flushing, intermittent headaches (cluster headaches), depression.

Aggravating or Relieving Factors

Relief by analgesics or sleep. Exacerbation by foods (chocolate, alcohol, wine, cheese, monosodium glutamate), emotional upset, menses; hypertension, trauma; lack of sleep; exacerbation by fatigue, exertion.

3. Medications

ACE inhibitors and antagonists, alpha-adrenergic blockers, metronidazole, calcium channel blockers, e.g., nifedipine, H_2-blockers, oral contraceptives, nitrates, NSAIDs, selective-serotonin reuptake inhibitors.

二、头　痛

1. 主　诉

55 岁女性，头痛 4 小时。

2. 现病史

疼痛性质（钝，带状，尖锐、搏动性），位置（眶后，颞部，枕下，双侧或单侧），典型头痛的发作时程；发作（逐渐或突然起病）；加重或缓解因素；一日中的时间，仰卧位的影响。头痛起病的年龄；严重程度，频率变化；是否睡眠中痛醒；镇痛药或可待因的使用；偏头痛家族史。"有史以来最严重的头痛"→ 蛛网膜下腔出血。

前驱症状：视觉盲点，视力模糊；恶心，呕吐，感觉障碍。

伴随症状：虚弱，复视，畏光，发烧，流鼻涕（鼻窦炎）；颈项强直（脑膜炎）；眼痛或眼红（青光眼）；共济失调，构音障碍，短暂性失明。流泪，潮红，间歇性头痛（丛集性头痛），抑郁。

加重或缓解因素：止痛药或睡眠缓解，食物（巧克力，酒精，葡萄酒，奶酪，味精）加重，情绪低落，月经；高血压，外伤；睡眠不足；疲劳、劳累加剧。

3. 药物史

血管紧张素转换酶抑制剂或受体拮抗剂，α-肾上腺素能阻滞剂，甲硝唑，钙通道阻滞剂，例如硝苯地平，H_2-阻滞剂，口服避孕药，硝酸盐，非甾体抗炎药，选择性 5-羟色胺再摄取抑制剂。

4. Physical Examination

General Appearance: Note whether the patient appears ill or well.

Vital Signs: BP (hypertension), pulse, temperature (fever), respiratory rate.

HEENT: Cranial or temporal tenderness (temporal arteritis), asymmetric pupil reactivity; papilledema, extraocular movements, visual field deficits. Conjunctival injection, lacrimation, rhinorrhea (cluster headache). Temporomandibular joint tenderness (TMJ syndrome); temporal or ocular bruits (arteriovenous malformation); sinus tenderness (sinusitis). Dental infection, tooth tenderness to percussion (abscess).

Neck: Neck rigidity ; paraspinal muscle tenderness.

Skin: Café au lait spots (neurofibromatosis), facial angiofibroma (adenoma sebaceum).

Neuro: Cranial nerve palsies (intracranial tumor); auditory acuity, focal weakness (intracranial tumor), sensory deficits, deep tendon reflexes, ataxia.

5. Labs

Electrolytes, ESR, MRI scan, lumbar puncture. CBC with differential.

Indications for MRI scan: Focal neurologic signs, papilledema, decreased visual acuity, increased frequency or severity of headache, excruciating or paroxysmal headache, awakening from sleep, persistent vomiting, head trauma with focal neurologic signs or lethargy.

6. Differential Diagnosis

Migraine, tension headache; systemic infection, subarachnoid hemorrhage, sinusitis, arteriovenous malformation, hypertensive encephalopathy, temporal arteritis, meningitis, encephalitis, post-concussion syndrome, intracranial tumor, venous sinus thrombosis, benign intracranial hypertension (pseudotumor cerebri), subdural hematoma, trigeminal neuralgia, glaucoma, analgesic overuse.

4. 体格检查

一般情况：注意对患者病情的一般印象。

生命体征：血压（高血压），脉搏，体温（发热），呼吸频率。

头眼耳鼻喉：颅骨或颞部压痛（颞动脉炎），瞳孔对光反射不对称；视乳头水肿，眼外肌运动，视野缺损。结膜充血，流泪，流涕（丛集性头痛）。颞下颌关节压痛（颞下颌关节综合征）；颞部或眼旁杂音（动静脉畸形）；鼻窦压痛（鼻窦炎）。牙齿感染，牙齿压痛（脓肿）。

颈部：颈部僵硬；椎旁肌压痛。

皮肤：咖啡色斑点（神经纤维瘤病），面部血管纤维瘤（皮脂腺瘤）。

神经系统：颅神经麻痹（颅内肿瘤），听觉敏锐度，局灶性无力（颅内肿瘤），感觉缺陷，深腱反射，共济失调。

5. 实验室检查

电解质，血沉，MRI，腰椎穿刺，血常规。

MRI 适应证：局灶性神经系统体征，视乳头水肿，视力下降，头痛的频率或严重度增加，剧烈或阵发性头痛，睡眠中痛醒，持续呕吐，具有局灶性神经系统体征或嗜睡的头部外伤。

6. 鉴别诊断

偏头痛，紧张性头痛；全身感染，蛛网膜下腔出血，鼻窦炎，动静脉畸形，高血压脑病，颞动脉炎，脑膜炎，脑炎，脑震荡后综合征，颅内肿瘤，静脉窦血栓形成，良性颅内高压症（假性颅内肿瘤），硬膜下血肿，三叉神经痛，青光眼，镇痛药过度使用。

Characteristics of Migraine: Childhood to early adult onset; family history of headache; aura of scotomas or scintillations, unilateral pulsating or throbbing pain; nausea, vomiting. Lasts 2-6 hours; relief with sleep.

Characteristics of Tension Headache: Bilateral, generalized, bitemporal or suboccipital. Band-like pressure; throbbing pain, occurs late in day; related to stress. Onset in adolescence or young adult. Lasts hours and is usually relieved by simple analgesics.

Characteristics of Cluster Headache: Unilateral, retroorbital searing pain, lacrimation, nasal and conjunctival congestion. Young males; lasts 20-60 min. Occurs several times each day over several weeks, followed by pain-free periods.

偏头痛的特征：儿童期至成年早期发病；头痛家族史；盲点或闪烁等先兆，单侧搏动或搏动性疼痛；恶心，呕吐。持续 2~6 小时；睡眠可缓解。

紧张性头痛的特征：双侧性，全身性，双侧颞部或枕部。带状压力感；抽搐的疼痛，发生在一天的靠后时间段；与压力有关。起病于青春期或年轻的成年人。持续数小时，一般镇痛药即可缓解。

丛集性头痛的特征：单侧，眶后灼痛，流泪，鼻和结膜充血。青年男性；持续 20~60 min。在数周内每天出现几次，然后进入无痛期。

三、胸痛（Chest Pain）

1. Chief Complaint

The patient is a 56-year-old Asian male with hypertension who complains of chest pain for 3 hours.

2. History of the Present Illness

Duration of chest pain. Location, radiation (to arm, jaw, back), character (squeezing, sharp, dull), intensity, rate of onset (gradually or suddenly); relationship of pain to activity (at rest, during sleep, during exercise); relief by nitroglycerine; increase in frequency or severity of baseline anginal pattern. Improvement or worsening of pain. Past episodes of chest pain. Age of onset of angina.

Associated Symptoms: Diaphoresis, nausea, vomiting, dyspnea, orthopnea, edema, palpitations, syncope, dysphagia, cough, sputum, paresthesia.

Aggravating and Relieving Factors: Effect of inspiration on pain; effect of eating, NSAIDS, alcohol, stress. Cardiac testing: Past stress testing, stress echocardiogram, angiogram, nuclear scans, ECGs. Cardiac risk factors: Hypertension, hyperlipidemia, diabetes, smoking, and a strong family history (coronary artery disease in early or mid-adulthood in a first-degree relative).

3. Past Medical History

History of diabetes, claudication, stroke. Exercise tolerance; history of peptic ulcer disease. Prior history of myocardial infarction, coronary bypass grafting or angioplasty.

4. Social History

Smoking, alcohol, cocaine usage, illicit drugs.

5. Medications

Aspirin, beta-blockers, estrogen.

三、胸　痛

1. 主　诉

56 岁亚裔男性高血压患者，胸痛 3 小时。

2. 现病史

胸痛持续时间。位置，辐射（手臂，下颌，背部），性质（挤压，尖锐，钝痛），强度，发病方式（逐渐或突然）；疼痛与活动的关系（休息，睡眠，运动期间）；硝酸甘油缓解；已患心绞痛加重的频率或程度。疼痛的改善或恶化因素。既往胸痛发作。心绞痛起病年龄。

伴随症状：出汗，恶心，呕吐，呼吸困难，端坐呼吸，水肿，心悸，晕厥，吞咽困难，咳嗽，咳痰，感觉异常。

加重和缓解因素：吸气对疼痛的影响；饮食，非甾体抗炎药，酒精，压力的影响。心脏检查：既往负荷试验，负荷超声心动图，血管造影，核素扫描，心电图。心脏危险因素：高血压，高血脂，糖尿病，吸烟、强家族史（一级亲属青年或中年患冠心病）。

3. 既往史

糖尿病，跛行，中风病史，运动耐力，消化性溃疡病史。既往心肌梗死，冠状动脉搭桥术或血管成形术。

4. 社会史

吸烟，饮酒，可卡因，非法药物。

5. 药物史

阿司匹林，β-受体阻滞剂，雌激素。

6. Physical Examination

General: Note whether the patient appears ill, well, or malnourished. Visible pain, apprehension, distress, pallor.

Vital Signs: Pulse (tachycardia or bradycardia), BP (hypertension or hypotension), respirations (tachypnea), temperature.

Skin: Cold extremities (peripheral vascular disease), xanthomas (familial hypercholesterolemia).

HEENT: Fundi, "silver wire" arteries, arteriolar narrowing, A-V nicking, hypertensive retinopathy; carotid bruits, jugular venous distention.

Chest: Inspiratory crackles (heart failure), percussion note.

Heart: Decreased intensity of first heart sound (S1) (LV dysfunction); third heart sound (S3 gallop) (heart failure, dilation), S4 gallop (more audible in the left lateral position; decreased LV compliance due to ischemia); systolic mitral insufficiency murmur (papillary muscle dysfunction), cardiac rub (pericarditis).

Abdomen: Hepatojugular reflux, epigastric tenderness, hepatomegaly, pulsatile mass (aortic aneurysm).

Rectal: Occult blood.

Extremities: Edema (heart failure), femoral bruits, unequal or diminished pulses (aortic dissection); calf pain, swelling (thrombosis).

Neurologic: Altered mental status.

7. Labs

Electrocardiographic Findings in Acute Myocardial Infarction: ST segment elevations in two contiguous leads with ST depressions in reciprocal leads, hyperacute T waves.

Chest X-ray: Cardiomegaly, pulmonary edema (CHF). Electrolytes, LDH, CBC. CPK with isoenzymes, troponin I or troponin T, myoglobin. Echocardiography.

6. 体格检查

一般情况：注意对患者病情的一般印象。明显的疼痛，忧虑，痛苦，面色苍白。

生命体征：脉搏（心动过速或心动过缓），血压（高血压或低血压），呼吸（呼吸急促），体温。

皮肤：四肢发冷（周围血管病），黄色瘤（家族性高胆固醇血症）。

头眼耳鼻喉：眼底，"银丝"动脉，小动脉变窄，动静脉压痕，高血压视网膜病；颈动脉杂音，颈静脉怒张。

胸部：吸气性湿啰音（心力衰竭），叩诊音。

心脏：第一心音（S1）强度变弱（左心功能不全）；第三心音（S3奔马律，心力衰竭），第四心音（S4 奔马律，左侧位更易闻及；系缺血导致左室顺应性降低）；收缩期二尖瓣关闭不全杂音（乳头肌功能障碍），心包摩擦音（心包炎）。

腹部：肝颈静脉反流征，上腹压痛，肝大，搏动性包块（主动脉瘤）。

直肠：隐血。

肢体：水肿（心力衰竭）；股动脉杂音，脉搏强弱不均或减弱（主动脉夹层）；小腿疼痛、肿胀（血栓）。

神经系统：精神状态改变。

7. 实验室检查

急性心梗的心电图：梗死部位连续两个导联 ST 段抬高，对应导联 ST 压低，超急性 T 波。

胸片：心脏增大，肺水肿（慢性心衰）。电解质，乳酸脱氢酶，血常规。肌酸肌酶及同工酶，肌钙蛋白 I 或 T，肌红蛋白。超声心动图。

8. Differential Diagnosis of Chest Pain

(1) Acute Pericarditis. Characterized by pleuritic-type chest pain and diffuse ST segment elevation.

(2) Aortic Dissection. "Tearing" chest pain with uncontrolled hypertension, widened mediastinum and increased aortic prominence on chest X-ray.

(3) Esophageal Rupture. Occurs after vomiting; X-ray may reveal air in mediastinum or a left side hydrothorax.

(4) Acute Cholecystitis. Characterized by right subcostal abdominal pain with anorexia, nausea, vomiting, and fever.

(5) Acute Peptic Ulcer Disease. Epigastric pain with melena or hematemesis, and anemia.

8. 胸痛鉴别诊断

（1）急性心包炎：以胸膜炎性胸痛和弥漫性 ST 段抬高为特征。

（2）主动脉夹层："撕裂"样胸痛伴未控制的高血压，胸片示纵隔增宽、主动脉突出。

（3）食管破裂：呕吐后发生，X 片可显示纵隔积气或左侧胸腔积液。

（4）急性胆囊炎：特征为右肋下疼痛，伴有厌食、恶心、呕吐和发热。

（5）急性消化性溃疡：上腹痛伴黑便、呕血或贫血。

四、腹痛（Abdominal Pain）

1. Chief Complaint

The patient is a 45-year-old male with diabetes who complains of right lower quadrant abdominal pain for 3 hours.

2. History of the Present Illness

Duration of pain, pattern of progression; exact location at onset and at present; diffuse or localized; character at onset and at present (burning, crampy, sharp, dull); constant or intermittent ("colicky"); radiation of pain (to shoulder, back, groin); sudden or gradual onset. Effect of eating, vomiting, defecation, flatus, urination, inspiration, movement, position on the pain. Timing and characteristics of last bowel movement. Similar episodes in the past; relation to the last menstrual period.

Associated Symptoms: Fever, chills, nausea, vomiting (bilious, feculent, blood, coffee ground-colored material); vomiting before or after onset of pain; jaundice, constipation, change in bowel habits or stool caliber, obstipation (inability to pass gas); chest pain, diarrhea, hematochezia (rectal bleeding), melena (black, tarry stools); dysuria, hematuria, anorexia, weight loss, dysphagia, odynophagia (painful swallowing); early satiety, trauma.

Aggravating or Relieving Factors: Fatty food intolerance, medications, aspirin, NSAIDs, narcotics, anticholinergics, laxatives, antacids.

3. Past Medical History

History of abdominal surgery (appendectomy, cholecystectomy), hernias, gallstones; coronary disease, kidney stones; alcoholism, cirrhosis, peptic ulcer, dyspepsia. Endoscopies, X-rays, upper GI series.

四、腹 痛

1. 主 诉

45 岁男性，糖尿病患者，右下腹痛 3 小时。

2. 现病史

疼痛持续时间，进展方式；起病时和目前的确切位置；弥漫性或局限性；起病时和现在的性质（灼热，痉挛，尖锐，钝痛）；持续性或间歇性（"绞痛"）；放射痛（肩部，背部，腹股沟）；突然或逐渐发作。进食，呕吐，解便，排气，排尿，吸气，运动，姿势对疼痛的影响。最后解便的时间和特点。既往类似发作；与末次月经的关系。

伴随症状：发热，发冷，恶心，呕吐（胆汁，浊臭，血液，咖啡样物质）；呕吐与疼痛的时间关系；黄疸，便秘，排便习惯或大便形状改变，便秘（无法排气）；胸痛，腹泻，便血（直肠出血），黑便（黑色柏油样）；排尿困难，血尿，厌食，体重减轻，吞咽困难，吞咽痛；早饱，外伤。

加重或缓解因素：脂肪食物不耐受，药物，阿司匹林，非甾体抗炎药，麻醉剂，抗胆碱能药，泻药，抗酸药。

3. 既往史

腹部手术史（阑尾切除术，胆囊切除术），疝气，胆结石；冠心病，肾结石；酗酒，肝硬化，消化性溃疡，消化不良。内窥镜检查，上消化道 X 射线检查。

4. Physical Examination

General Appearance: Note whether the patient appears ill, well, or malnourished. Degree of distress, body positioning to relieve pain, nutritional status. Signs of dehydration, septic appearance.

Vitals: Temperature (fever), pulse (tachycardia), BP (hypotension), respiratory rate (tachypnea).

HEENT: Pale conjunctiva, scleral icterus, atherosclerotic retinopathy, "silver wire" arteries; flat neck veins (hypovolemia). Lymphadenopathy, Virchow node (left supraclavicular mass).

Abdomen

Inspection: Scars, ecchymosis, visible peristalsis (small bowel obstruction), distension. Scaphoid, flat.

Auscultation: Absent bowel sounds (paralytic ileus or late obstruction), high-pitched rushes (obstruction), bruits (ischemic colitis).

Palpation: Begin palpation in quadrant diagonally opposite to point of maximal pain with patient's legs flexed and relaxed. Bimanual palpation of flank (renal disease). Rebound tenderness; hepatomegaly, splenomegaly, masses; hernias (incisional, inguinal, femoral). Pulsating masses; costovertebral angle tenderness. Bulging flanks, shifting dullness, fluid wave (ascites).

Specific Signs on Palpation

Murphy's sign: Inspiratory arrest with right upper quadrant palpation → cholecystitis.

Charcot's sign: Right upper quadrant pain, jaundice, fever → gallstones.

Courvoisier's sign: Palpable, nontender gallbladder with jaundice → pancreatic malignancy.

McBurney's point tenderness: Located two thirds of the way between umbilicus and right anterior superior iliac spine → appendicitis.

4. 体格检查

一般情况：注意对患者病情的一般印象。痛苦程度，缓解疼痛的体位，营养状况。脱水征，败血症外观。

生命体征：体温（发热），脉搏（心动过速），血压（低血压），呼吸频率（心动过速）。

头眼耳鼻喉：结膜苍白，巩膜黄染，动脉粥样硬化性视网膜病变，"银丝"动脉；颈静脉扁平（血容量不足）。淋巴结肿大，魏尔啸淋巴结（左锁骨上淋巴结）。

腹部：

视诊：疤痕，瘀斑，可见肠蠕动（小肠梗阻），膨隆，舟状腹，扁平腹。

听诊：肠鸣音消失（麻痹性肠梗阻或晚期梗阻），高调的气过水声（梗阻），杂音（缺血性结肠炎）。

触诊：患者屈腿放松，从最重疼痛点对侧象限开始触诊。双手触诊胁腹（肾脏疾病）。反跳痛；肝大，脾大，肿块；疝气（切口疝，腹股沟疝，股疝）。搏动性包块，肋脊角压痛。腹侧壁膨出，移动性浊音，波动感（腹水）。

触诊特殊体征：

Murphy 氏征：右上腹触诊时停止吸气 → 胆囊炎。

Charcot 氏征：右上腹痛伴黄疸及发热 → 胆结石。

Courvoisier 体征：可触及的无痛性胆囊伴黄疸 → 胰腺恶性肿瘤。

McBurney 压痛点：由脐向右髂前上棘连线距离的 2/3 处 → 阑尾炎

Iliopsoas sign: Elevation of legs against examiner's hand causes pain → retrocecal appendicitis.

Obturator sign: Flexion of right thigh and external rotation of thigh causes pain in pelvic appendicitis.

Rovsing's sign: Manual pressure and release at left lower quadrant colon causes referred pain at McBurney's point → appendicitis.

Cullen's sign: Bluish periumbilical discoloration → peritoneal hemorrhage.

Grey Turner's sign: Flank ecchymosis → retroperitoneal hemorrhage.

Percussion: Loss of liver dullness (perforated viscus, free air in peritoneum); liver and spleen span by percussion.

Rectal Examination: Masses, tenderness, impacted stool; gross or occult blood.

Genital/Pelvic Examination: Cervical discharge, adnexal tenderness, uterine size, masses, cervical motion tenderness.

Extremities: Femoral pulses, popliteal pulses, edema.

Skin: Jaundice, dependent purpura (mesenteric infarction), petechia (gonococcemia).

Stigmata of Liver Disease: Spider angiomata, periumbilical collateral veins (Caput medusae), gynecomastia, ascites, hepatosplenomegaly, testicular atrophy.

5. Labs

CBC, electrolytes, liver function tests, amylase, lipase, UA, pregnancy test. ECG.

Chest X-ray: Free air under diaphragm, infiltrates, effusion (pancreatitis).

X-rays of abdomen (acute abdomen series): Subdiaphragmatic free air, distended loops of bowel, sentinel loop, air fluid levels, thumb printing, calcifications, fecaliths.

髂腰肌征：抬高腿抵抗检查者的手导致疼痛 → 盲肠阑尾炎。

闭孔肌征：右大腿屈曲外旋导致疼痛 → 骨盆阑尾炎。

Rovsing 氏征：徒手压迫左下象限结肠突然释放导致 McBurney 点牵涉痛 → 阑尾炎。

Cullen 氏征：脐周腹部皮肤蓝染 → 腹腔内出血。

Grey Turner 氏征：两侧胁腹部瘀斑 → 腹膜后出血。

叩诊：肝浊音界消失（内脏穿孔，腹腔内游离气体）；肝界和脾界。

直肠检查：肿物，压痛，粪便嵌塞；明显便血或潜血。

生殖器/盆腔检查：宫颈分泌物，附件压痛，子宫大小，肿块，宫颈活动痛。

四肢：股动脉搏动，腘动脉搏动，水肿。

皮肤：黄疸，继发性紫癜（肠系膜梗死），瘀点（淋球菌血症）。

肝病体征：蜘蛛痣，脐周静脉曲张（海蛇头），男性乳房发育，腹水，肝脾肿大，睾丸萎缩。

5. 实验室检查

血常规，电解质，肝功能检查，淀粉酶，脂肪酶，尿常规，妊娠试验。心电图。

胸片：横膈膜下游离气体，浸润，积液（胰腺炎）。

腹部 X 片（急腹症）：膈下游离气体，肠胀环，哨兵攀征，气液平，拇指印，钙化，粪便。

6. Differential Diagnosis

Generalized Pain: Intestinal infarction, peritonitis, obstruction, diabetic ketoacidosis, acute porphyria, penetrating posterior duodenal ulcer, psychogenic pain.

Right Upper Quadrant: Cholecystitis, cholangitis, hepatitis, gastritis, pancreatitis, hepatic metastases, retrocecal appendicitis, pneumonia, peptic ulcer.

Epigastrium: Gastritis, peptic ulcer, gastroesophageal reflux disease, esophagitis, gastroenteritis, pancreatitis, perforated viscus, ileus, myocardial infarction, aortic aneurysm.

Left Upper Quadrant: Peptic ulcer, gastritis, esophagitis, gastroesophageal reflux, pancreatitis, myocardial ischemia, pneumonia, splenic infarction, pulmonary embolus.

Left Lower Quadrant: Diverticulitis, intestinal obstruction, colitis, strangulated hernia, inflammatory bowel disease, gastroenteritis, pyelonephritis, nephrolithiasis, mesenteric lymphadenitis, mesenteric thrombosis, aortic aneurysm, volvulus, intussusception, salpingitis, ovarian cyst, ectopic pregnancy, endometriosis, testicular torsion, psychogenic pain.

Right Lower Quadrant: Appendicitis, diverticulitis, salpingitis, endometritis, endometriosis, intussusception, ectopic pregnancy, hemorrhage or rupture of ovarian cyst, renal calculus.

Pelvic: Cystitis, salpingitis, ectopic pregnancy, diverticulitis, strangulated hernia, endometriosis, appendicitis, ovarian cyst torsion; bladder distension, nephrolithiasis, prostatitis, malignancy.

6. 鉴别诊断

全腹性疼痛：肠梗死，腹膜炎，梗阻，糖尿病性酮症酸中毒，急性卟啉症，十二指肠后壁穿透性溃疡，精神性疼痛。

右上象限：胆囊炎，胆管炎，肝炎，胃炎，胰腺炎，肝转移瘤，盲肠阑尾炎，肺炎，消化性溃疡。

上腹部：胃炎，消化性溃疡，胃食管反流病，食管炎，肠胃炎，胰腺炎，内脏穿孔，肠梗阻，心肌梗死，主动脉瘤。

左上象限：消化性溃疡，胃炎，食管炎，胃食管反流，胰腺炎，心肌缺血，肺炎，脾梗死，肺栓塞。

左下象限：憩室炎，肠梗阻，结肠炎，绞窄性疝，炎性肠病，胃肠炎，肾盂肾炎，肾结石病，肠系膜淋巴结炎，肠系膜血栓形成、主动脉瘤、肠扭转、肠套叠、输卵管炎、卵巢囊肿、异位妊娠、子宫内膜异位症，睾丸扭转，精神性疼痛。

右下腹：阑尾炎，憩室炎，输卵管炎，子宫内膜炎，子宫内膜异位，肠套叠，异位妊娠，卵巢囊肿出血或破裂，肾结石。

盆腔：膀胱炎，输卵管炎，异位妊娠，憩室炎，绞窄性疝，子宫内膜异位症，阑尾炎，卵巢囊肿扭转；膀胱膨胀，肾结石，前列腺炎，恶性肿瘤。

五、心悸（Palpitations）

1. Chief Complaint

The patient is a 70-year-old white male with hypertension who complains of palpitations for 8 hours.

2. History of the Present Illness

Palpitations (rapid or irregular heart beat), fatigue, dizziness, nausea, dyspnea, edema; duration of palpitations. Results of previous ECGs.

Associated Symptoms: Chest pain, pleuritic pain, syncope, fatigue, exercise intolerance, diaphoresis, symptoms of hyperthyroidism (tremor, anxiety).

Cardiac History: Hypertension, coronary disease, rheumatic heart disease, arrhythmias.

3. Past Medical History

Diabetes, pneumonia, noncompliance with cardiac medications, pericarditis, hyperthyroidism, electrolyte abnormalities, COPD, mitral valve stenosis; diet pills, decongestants, alcohol, caffeine, cocaine.

4. Physical Examination

General Appearance: Note whether the patient appears ill, well, or malnourished. Respiratory distress, anxiety, diaphoresis. Dyspnea, pallor.

Vital Signs: BP (hypotension), pulse (irregular tachycardia), respiratory rate, temperature.

HEENT: Retinal hemorrhages (emboli), jugular venous distention, carotid bruits; thyromegaly (hyperthyroidism).

Chest: Crackles (rales).

Heart: Irregular rhythm (atrial fibrillation); dyskinetic apical pulse, displaced point of maximal impulse (cardiomegaly), S4, mitral regurgitation murmur (rheumatic fever); pericardial rub (pericarditis).

五、心　悸

1. 主　诉

70 岁白人男性，高血压患者，心悸 8 小时。

2. 现病史

心悸（快速或不规则心跳），疲劳，头晕，恶心，呼吸困难，水肿；心悸持续的时间。既往心电图结果。

伴随症状：胸痛，胸膜炎疼痛，晕厥，疲劳，运动不耐受，发汗，甲亢症状（震颤，焦虑）。

心脏病史：高血压，冠心病，风湿性心脏病，心律不齐。

3. 既往史

糖尿病，肺炎，心脏病药物依从性差，心包炎，甲亢，电解质异常，慢性阻塞性肺疾病，二尖瓣狭窄；减肥药，缓解充血药，酒精，咖啡因，可卡因。

4. 体格检查

一般情况：注意对患者病情的一般印象。呼吸窘迫，焦虑，发汗。呼吸困难，面色苍白。

生命体征：BP（低血压），脉搏（不规则心动过速），呼吸频率，体温。

头眼耳鼻喉：视网膜出血（栓子），颈静脉怒张，颈动脉杂音；甲状腺肿大（甲亢）。

胸部：啰音。

心脏：心律不齐（房颤）；心尖搏动障碍，最强心尖搏动点移位（心脏肥大），S4，二尖瓣反流性杂音（风湿热）；心包摩擦音（心包炎）。

Rectal: Occult blood.

Extremities: Peripheral pulses with irregular timing and amplitude. Edema, cyanosis, petechia (emboli). Femoral artery bruits (atherosclerosis).

Neuro: Altered mental status, motor weakness (embolic stroke), CN 2-12, sensory; dysphasia, dysarthria (stroke); tremor (hyperthyroidism).

5. Labs

Sodium, potassium, BUN, creatinine; magnesium; drug levels; CBC; serial cardiac enzymes; CPK, LDH, TSH, free T4. Chest X-ray.

ECG: Irregular baseline with irregular R-R intervals without P waves, rapid fibrillary waves (320 per minute) with the ventricular response rate 130-180 per minute (atrial fibrillation).

Echocardiogram for cardiac chamber size.

6. Differential Diagnosis of Atrial Fibrillation

Lone Atrial Fibrillation: No underlying disease state.

Cardiac Causes: Hypertensive heart disease with left ventricular hypertrophy, heart failure, mitral valve stenosis or regurgitation, pericarditis, hypertrophic cardiomyopathy, coronary artery disease, myocardial infarction, aortic stenosis, amyloidosis.

Noncardiac Causes: Hypoglycemia, theophylline intoxication, pneumonia, asthma, chronic obstructive pulmonary disease, pulmonary embolism, heavy alcohol intake or alcohol withdrawal, hyperthyroidism, systemic illness, electrolyte abnormalities. Stimulant abuse, excessive caffeine, over-the-counter cold remedies, illicit drugs.

直肠：隐血。

肢体：外周脉搏不规律、幅度不一。水肿，发绀，瘀点（栓子），股动脉杂音（动脉粥样硬化）。

神经系统：精神状态改变，运动无力（脑栓塞），颅神经 2-12，感官；吞咽困难，构音障碍（中风），震颤（甲亢）。

5. 实验室检查

钠，钾，尿素氮，肌酐；镁；药物水平；血常规；心肌酶谱；血清磷酸激酶同工酶，乳酸脱氢酶，促甲状腺激素，游离甲状腺素 4。胸片。

ECG：P 波消失，基线不规则，R-R 间期不规则，伴快速纤颤波（320 次/分），心室率是 130～180 次/分 → 房颤。

超声心动图：评估房室大小。

6. 房颤鉴别诊断

孤立性房颤：无潜在的疾病。

心源性：伴有左心室肥大，心脏衰竭，二尖瓣狭窄或反流的高血压心脏病，心包炎，肥厚型心肌病，冠状动脉疾病，心肌梗死，主动脉瓣狭窄，淀粉样变性。

非心源性：低血糖，茶碱中毒，肺炎，哮喘，慢性阻塞性肺疾病，肺栓塞，大量饮酒或戒酒，甲亢，全身性疾病，电解质异常。兴奋剂滥用，咖啡因过量，非处方感冒药，违禁药物。

六、高血压（Hypertension）

1. Chief Complaint

The patient is a 56-year-old white male with coronary heart disease who presents with a blood pressure of 190/120 mmHg for 1 day.

2. History of the Present Illness

Degree of blood pressure elevation; patient's baseline BP from records; baseline BUN and creatinine. Age of onset of hypertension.

Associated Symptoms: Chest or back pain (aortic dissection), dyspnea, orthopnea, dizziness, blurred vision (hypertensive retinopathy); nausea, vomiting, headache (pheochromocytoma); lethargy, confusion (encephalopathy). Paroxysms of tremor, palpitations, diaphoresis; edema, thyroid disease, angina; flank pain, dysuria, pyelonephritis. Alcohol withdrawal, noncompliance with antihypertensives (clonidine or beta-blocker withdrawal), excessive salt, alcohol.

3. Medications

Over-the-counter cold remedies, beta-agonists, diet pills, eye medications (sympathomimetics), bronchodilators, cocaine, amphetamines, nonsteroidal anti-inflammatory agents, oral contraceptives, corticosteroids.

4. Past Medical History

Cardiac risk factors: Family history of coronary artery disease before age 55, diabetes, hypertension, smoking, hypercholesterolemia.

Past Testing: Urinalysis, ECG, creatinine.

5. Physical Examination

General Appearance: Delirium, confusion (hypertensive encephalopathy).

Vital Signs: Supine and upright blood pressure; BP in all extremities; pulse, temperature, respirations.

六、高血压

1. 主诉

56 岁白人男性，冠心病患者，血压 190/120 mmHg，持续 1 天。

2. 现病史

最高血压水平，有记录的基础血压水平，基础尿素氮和肌酐，起病年龄。

伴随症状：胸痛或背痛（主动脉夹层），呼吸困难，端坐呼吸，头晕，视力模糊（高血压性视网膜病）；恶心，呕吐，头痛（嗜铬细胞瘤）；嗜睡，意识模糊（脑病）。阵发性震颤，心悸，出汗；水肿，甲状腺疾病，心绞痛；腰痛，排尿困难，肾盂肾炎。酒精戒断，服用降压药依从性差（可乐定或 β-受体阻滞剂停药），盐摄入过量，酒精。

3. 药物史

非处方感冒药，β-受体激动剂，减肥药，眼药（拟交感神经药），支气管扩张药，可卡因，苯丙胺，非甾体抗炎药，口服避孕药，皮质类固醇。

4. 既往史

危险因素：早发冠心病家族史（55 岁前），糖尿病，高血压，吸烟，高胆固醇血症。

既往检查：尿常规，心电图，肌酐。

5. 体格检查

一般情况：谵妄，意识模糊（高血压脑病）。

生命体征：卧位和直立位血压；四肢血压；脉搏，体温，呼吸。

HEENT: Hypertensive retinopathy, hemorrhages, exudates, "cotton wool" spots, A-V nicking; papilledema; thyromegaly (hyperthyroidism). jugular venous distention, carotid bruits.

Chest: Crackles (rales, pulmonary edema), wheeze, intercostal bruits (aortic coarctation).

Heart: Rhythm; laterally displaced apical impulse with patient in left lateral position (ventricular hypertrophy); narrowly split S2 with increased aortic component; systolic ejection murmurs.

Abdomen: Renal bruits (bruit just below costal margin, renal artery stenosis); abdominal aortic enlargement (aortic aneurysm), renal masses, enlarged kidney (polycystic kidney disease); costovertebral angle tenderness. Truncal obesity (Cushing's syndrome).

Skin: Striae (Cushing's syndrome), uremic frost (chronic renal failure), hirsutism (adrenal hyperplasia), plethora (pheochromocytoma).

Extremities: Asymmetric femoral to radial pulses (coarctation of aortic); femoral bruits, edema; tremor (pheochromocytoma, hyperthyroidism).

Neuro: Altered mental status, rapid return phase of deep tendon reflexes (hyperthyroidism), localized weakness (stroke), visual acuity.

6. Labs

Potassium, BUN, creatinine, glucose, uric acid, CBC. UA with microscopic (RBC casts, hematuria, proteinuria). 24-hour urine for metanephrine, plasma catecholamines (pheochromocytoma), plasma renin activity.

12 Lead ECG: Evidence of ischemic heart disease, rhythm and conduction disturbances, or left ventricular hypertrophy.

Chest X-ray: Cardiomegaly, indentation of aorta (coarctation).

头眼耳鼻喉：高血压视网膜病变，出血，渗出，"棉绒"斑点，动静脉压痕；视乳头水肿；甲状腺肿大（甲亢）。颈静脉怒张，颈动脉杂音。

胸部：啰音（肺水肿），喘鸣，肋间杂音（主动脉缩窄）。

心脏：心律；患者左侧卧位触及心尖搏动移位（心室肥大）； S2变窄并分裂，主动脉成分增加；收缩期喷射样杂音。

腹部：肾脏杂音（杂音位于肋缘下，肾动脉狭窄）；腹主动脉扩张（主动脉瘤），肾脏肿块，肾脏增大（多囊肾）；肋脊角压痛。躯干型肥胖（库欣综合征）。

皮肤：皮纹（库欣综合征），尿毒症霜（慢性肾功能衰竭），多毛症（肾上腺增生），多血症（嗜铬细胞瘤）。

肢体：股动脉和桡动脉脉搏不对称（主动脉缩窄），股动脉杂音，水肿，震颤（嗜铬细胞瘤，甲亢）。

神经系统：精神状态改变，深肌腱反射亢进（甲亢），局部无力（中风），视力。

6. 实验室检查

钾，尿素氮，肌酐，葡萄糖，尿酸，血常规。 尿常规镜检（红细胞管型，血尿，蛋白尿）。24 小时尿肾上腺素，血浆儿茶酚胺（嗜铬细胞瘤），血浆肾素活性。

12 导心电图：缺血性心脏病，心律和传导障碍或左心室肥大的证据。

胸片：心脏肥大，主动脉压痕（缩窄）

7. Differential Diagnosis of Hypertension

(1) Primary (essential) Hypertension **(90%)**

(2) Secondary Hypertension: Renovascular hypertension, pheochromocytoma, cocaine use; withdrawal from alpha2 stimulants, clonidine or beta-blockers, alcohol withdrawal; noncompliance with antihypertensive medications.

Findings Suggesting Secondary Hypertension:

(1) Primary Aldosteronism: **Serum potassium <3.5 mmol/L while not taking medication.**

(2) Aortic Coarctation: **Femoral pulse delayed later than radial pulse; posterior systolic bruits below ribs.**

(3) Pheochromocytoma: **Tachycardia, tremor, pallor.**

(4) Renovascular Stenosis: **Paraumbilical abdominal bruits.**

(5) Polycystic Kidneys: **Flank or abdominal mass.**

(6) Pyelonephritis: **Urinary tract infections, costovertebral angle tenderness.**

(7) Renal Parenchymal Disease: **Increased serum creatinine, proteinuria.**

7. 高血压鉴别诊断

（1）原发性高血压（90%）

（2）继发性高血压：肾血管性高血压，嗜铬细胞瘤，可卡因的使用；α2 兴奋剂停药，可乐定或 β-受体阻滞剂，戒酒；服用降压药依从性差。

继发性高血压：

（1）原发性醛固酮增多症：未服用药物时血清钾<3.5 mmol/L。

（2）主动脉缩窄：股动脉脉搏晚于桡动脉，背部闻及收缩期杂音。

（3）嗜铬细胞瘤：心动过速，震颤，苍白。

（4）肾血管狭窄：脐旁腹部杂音。

（5）多囊肾：胁腹或腹部肿块。

（6）肾盂肾炎：尿路感染，肋脊角压痛。

（7）肾实质疾病：血清肌酐升高，蛋白尿。

七、晕厥 (Syncope)

1. Chief Complaint

The patient is a 63-year-old male with hypertension who presents with loss of consciousness for 1 minute, 1 hour before admission.

2. History of the Present Illness

Time of occurrence and description of the episode. Duration of unconsciousness, rate of onset; activity before and after event. Body position, arm position (reaching), neck position (turning to side), mental status before and after the event. Precipitants (fear, tension, hunger, pain, cough, micturition, defecation, exertion, Valsalva, hyperventilation, tight shirt collar). Seizure activity (tonic/clonic). Chest pain, palpitations, dyspnea, weakness. Post-syncopal disorientation, confusion, vertigo, flushing; urinary of fecal incontinence, tongue biting. Rate of return to alertness (delayed or spontaneous). Prodromal Symptoms: Nausea, diaphoresis, pallor, lightheadedness, dimming vision (vasovagal syncope).

3. Past Medical History

Past episodes of syncope, stroke, transient ischemic attacks, seizures, cardiac disease, arrhythmias, diabetes, anxiety attacks.

Past Testing: 24-hour Holter, exercise testing, cardiac testing, ECG, EEG.

4. Physical Examination

General Appearance: Note whether the patient appears ill or well. Level of alertness, respiratory distress, anxiety, diaphoresis. Dyspnea, pallor.

Vital Signs: Temperature, respiratory rate, pulse, postural vitals (supine and after standing 2 minutes). Blood pressure in all extremities; asymmetric radial to femoral artery pulsations (aortic dissection).

七、晕 厥

1. 主 诉

63 岁男性，高血压患者，入院前 1 小时意识丧失 1 分钟。

2. 现病史

发生的时间和发作的情况。持续失去意识的时间，发病频率；发作前后的活动。身体位置，手臂位置（伸直），颈部位置（转向一侧），发作前后的精神状态。诱发因素（恐惧，紧张，饥饿，疼痛，咳嗽，排尿，排便，劳累，Valsalva 动作，过度换气，衣领过紧）。癫痫发作（强直/阵挛）。胸痛，心悸，呼吸困难，虚弱。晕厥后定向障碍，意识模糊，眩晕，潮红；大小便失禁，舌咬伤。警觉恢复的速度（延迟或自发）。前驱症状：恶心，发汗，面色苍白，头昏眼花，视力减退（迷走性晕厥）。

3. 既往史

既往晕厥，中风，短暂性脑缺血发作，癫痫发作，心脏病，心律不齐，糖尿病，焦虑发作。

既往检查：24 小时动态心电图，运动试验，心脏检查，心电图，脑电图。

4. 体格检查

一般情况：注意对患者病情的一般印象。警觉性，呼吸窘迫，焦虑，发汗。呼吸困难，面色苍白。

生命体征：体温，呼吸频率，脉搏，仰卧和站立 2 分钟后的生命体征。四肢血压；桡动脉股动脉搏动不对称（主动脉夹层）。

HEENT: Cranial bruising (trauma). Pupil size and reactivity, extraocular movements; tongue or buccal lacerations (seizure); flat jugular veins (volume depletion); carotid or vertebral arteries bruits.

Skin: Pallor, turgor, capillary refill.

Chest: Crackles, rhonchi (aspiration).

Heart: Irregular rhythm (atrial fibrillation); systolic murmurs (aortic stenosis), friction rub.

Abdomen: Bruits, tenderness, pulsatile mass.

Genitourinary/Rectal: Occult blood, urinary or fecal incontinence (seizure).

Extremities: Needle marks, injection site fat atrophy (diabetes), extremity palpation for trauma.

Neuro: Cranial nerves 2-12, strength, gait, sensory, altered mental status; nystagmus. Turn the patient's head side to side, up and down; have the patient reach above head, and pick up the object.

5. Labs

ECG: Arrhythmias, conduction blocks. Chest X-ray, electrolytes, glucose, Mg, Bun, creatinine, CBC; 24-hour Holter monitor.

6. Differential Diagnosis

Non-cardiovascular Syncope

Metabolic: Hyperventilation, hypoglycemia, hypoxia.

Neurologic: Cerebrovascular insufficiency, normal pressure hydrocephalus, seizure, subclavian steal syndrome, increased intracranial pressure.

Psychiatric: Hysteria, major depression.

Cardiovascular Syncope

Reflex (heart structurally normal): Vasovagal, situational, cough, defecation, micturition, postprandial, sneeze, swallow, carotid sinus syncope.

头眼耳鼻喉：头部擦伤（创伤）。瞳孔大小和反应，眼外肌运动；舌或颊裂伤（癫痫发作）；颈静脉扁平（容量减少）；颈动脉或椎动脉杂音。

皮肤：苍白，弹性，毛细血管再充盈。

胸部：湿啰音，干啰音（呼气）。

心脏：心律不齐（房颤）；收缩期杂音（主动脉瓣狭窄），摩擦音。

腹部：杂音，压痛，搏动性包块。

泌尿生殖系统/直肠：潜血，尿或大便失禁（癫痫发作）。

四肢：针痕，注射部位脂肪萎缩（糖尿病），若有外伤触诊四肢。

神经系统：颅神经 2-12，力量，步态，感觉，精神状态改变；眼球震颤。上下左右旋转患者的头部；让患者伸臂过头，然后附身拾物。

5. 实验室检查

心电图：心律不齐，传导阻滞。胸片，电解质，葡萄糖，镁，尿素氮，肌酐，血常规；24 小时动态心电图。

6. 鉴别诊断

非心血管晕厥

代谢性：换气过度，低血糖，缺氧。

神经系统疾病：脑血管功能不全，正常颅压性脑积水，癫痫发作，锁骨下盗窃综合征，颅内压增高。

精神科：歇斯底里症，严重抑郁症。

心血管晕厥

反射性（心脏结构正常）：迷走神经性，情境性，咳嗽，排便，排尿，餐后，打喷嚏，吞咽，颈动脉窦晕厥。

Cardiac: Obstructive, aortic dissection, aortic stenosis, cardiac tamponade, hypertrophic cardiomyopathy, left ventricular dysfunction, myocardial infarction, myxoma, pulmonary embolism, pulmonary hypertension, pulmonary stenosis, arrhythmias, bradyarrhythmias, sick sinus syndrome, pacemaker failure, supraventricular and ventricular tachyarrhythmias.

Orthostatic hypotension.

Drug-induced.

心源性：阻塞性，主动脉夹层，主动脉瓣狭窄，心包填塞，肥厚型心肌病，左心功能不全，心肌梗死，黏液瘤，肺栓塞，肺动脉高压，肺动脉狭窄，心律失常，缓慢性心律失常，病态窦房结综合征，起搏器衰竭，室上性或室性心律失常。

　　直立性低血压。

　　药物源性。

八、呼吸困难（Dyspnea）

1. Chief Complaint

The patient is a 69-year-old female with hypertension who complains of shortness of breath for 6 hours.

2. History of the Present Illness

Rate of onset of shortness of breath (gradual, sudden), orthopnea (dyspnea when supine), paroxysmal nocturnal dyspnea (PND), chest pain, palpitations. Dyspnea with physical exertion; history of myocardial infarction, syncope. Past episodes; aggravating or relieving factors (noncompliance with medications, salt overindulgence). Edema, weight gain, cough, sputum, fever, anxiety; hemoptysis, leg pain (DVT).

3. Past Medical History

Emphysema, heart failure, hypertension, coronary artery disease, asthma, occupational exposures, HIV risk factors. Medications: Bronchodilators, cardiac medications (noncompliance), drug allergies.

Past Investigation: Cardiac testing, chest X-rays, ECG's, spirometry.

4. Physical Examination

General Appearance: Note whether the patient appears ill, well, or in distress. Respiratory distress, dyspnea, pallor, diaphoresis. Fluid input and output balance.

Vital Signs: BP (supine and upright), pulse (tachycardia), temperature, respiratory rate (tachypnea).

HEENT: jugular venous distention at 45 degrees, tracheal deviation (pneumothorax).

Chest: Stridor (foreign body), wheezing, crackles (rales); dullness to percussion (pleural effusion), barrel chest (COPD); unilateral hyperresonance (pneumothorax).

八、呼吸困难

1. 主　诉

69 岁女性，高血压，呼吸困难 6 小时。

2. 现病史

呼吸困难（逐渐起病，突然发生），端坐呼吸（仰卧时呼吸困难），夜间阵发性呼吸困难，胸痛，心悸，劳力性呼吸困难，心肌梗死史，晕厥史。既往发病；加重或缓解因素（服药依从性差，食盐量过多），水肿，体重增加，咳嗽，痰，发烧，焦虑；咯血，腿痛（深静脉血栓）。

3. 既往史

肺气肿，心力衰竭，高血压，冠状动脉疾病，哮喘，职业暴露，HIV 危险因素。药物：支气管扩张药，心脏药物（依从性差），药物过敏。

既往检查：心脏检查，胸部 X 光检查，心电图，肺活量测定。

4. 体格检查

一般情况：注意对患者病情的一般印象。呼吸窘迫，呼吸困难，面色苍白，出汗。液体出入量平衡。

生命体征：血压（仰卧和直立），脉搏（心动过速），体温，呼吸频率（呼吸急促）。

头眼耳鼻喉：45 度颈静脉怒张，气管移位（气胸）。

胸部：喘鸣（异物），喘息，啰音，叩诊浊音（胸腔积液），桶状胸（慢性阻塞性肺病）；单侧过清音（气胸）。

Heart: Lateral displacement of point of maximal impulse; irregular rate, irregular rhythm (atrial fibrillation); S3 gallop (LV dilation), S4 (myocardial infarction), holosystolic apex murmur (mitral regurgitation); faint heart sounds (pericardial effusion).

Abdomen: Abdominojugular reflux (pressing on abdomen increases jugular vein distention), hepatomegaly, liver tenderness.

Extremities: Edema, pulses, cyanosis, clubbing finger. Calf tenderness or swelling (DVT).

Neurologic: Altered mental status.

5. Labs

ABG, cardiac enzymes; chest X-ray (cardiomegaly, hyperinflation with flattened diaphragms, infiltrates, effusions, pulmonary edema), ventilation/perfusion scan.

Electrocardiogram:

(1) ST segment depression or elevation, new left bundle-branch block.

(2) ST elevations in two contiguous leads, with ST depressions in reciprocal leads (MI).

6. Differential Diagnosis

Heart failure, myocardial infarction, upper airway obstruction, pneumonia, pulmonary embolism, chronic obstructive pulmonary disease, asthma, pneumothorax, foreign body aspiration, hyperventilation, malignancy, anemia.

心脏：最强心尖搏动点横向移位；不规则频率，不规则的节律（心房颤动）；S3 奔马律（左心室扩张），S4 奔马律（心肌梗死），全收缩期心尖杂音（二尖瓣关闭不全）；心音低钝（心包积液）。

腹部：腹颈静脉反流征（按压腹部会加重颈静脉怒张），肝大，肝脏触痛。

肢体：水肿，脉搏，发绀，杵状指。小腿压痛或肿胀（深静血栓）。

神经系统：精神状态改变。

5. 实验室检查

动脉血气分析，心肌酶谱；胸片（心脏增大，过度充气伴横膈膜平直，浸润，积液，肺水肿），通气/灌注扫描。

心电图：

（1）ST 段压低或抬高，新发左束支传导阻滞。

（2）相邻两导连 ST 段抬高，镜像导连 ST 段压低（心肌梗死）。

6. 鉴别诊断

心力衰竭，心肌梗死，上呼吸道阻塞，肺炎，肺栓塞，慢性阻塞性肺疾病，哮喘，气胸，异物吸入，过度换气，恶性肿瘤，贫血。

九、喘息（Wheezing）

1. Chief Complaint

The patient is a 60-year-old male with hypertension who complains of wheezing for one day.

2. History of the Present Illness

Onset, duration, and progression of wheezing; severity of attack compared to previous episodes; cough, fever, chills, purulent sputum. Frequency of bronchodilator use, relief of symptoms by bronchodilators. Frequency of exacerbations and hospitalizations or emergency department visits; duration of past exacerbations, steroid dependency, history of intubation, home oxygen or nebulizer use. Precipitating factors, exposure to allergens (foods, pollen, animals, drugs); seasons that provoke symptoms; exacerbation by exercise, aspirin, beta-blockers, recent upper respiratory infection; chest pain, foreign body aspiration. Worsening at night or with infection. Treatment given in emergency room and response.

3. Past Medical History

Previous episodes of asthma, COPD, pneumonia. Baseline arterial blood gas results; past pulmonary function testing.

4. Family History

Family history of asthma, allergies, hay fever, atopic dermatitis.

5. Social History

Smoking, alcohol.

6. Physical Examination

General Appearance: Note whether the patient appears cachectic, well, or in distress. Dyspnea, respiratory distress, diaphoresis, somnolence, anxiety, pallor.

九、喘　息

1. 主　诉

60 岁男性，高血压患者，喘息 1 天。

2. 现病史

喘息起病，持续时间和进展；较前相比的严重程度；咳嗽，发烧，寒战，脓痰。支气管扩张剂用药频率，支气管扩张剂可否减轻症状。加重、住院或急诊的频率；既往发作的持续时间，类固醇依赖性，插管史，家庭吸氧或使用雾化器。诱发因素，接触过敏原（食物，花粉，动物，药物）；症状易发的季节；运动，阿司匹林，β-受体阻滞剂，近期上呼吸道感染史；胸痛，异物吸入。晚上或感染时症状加重。急诊室接受治疗及疗效。

3. 既往史

既往哮喘，慢性阻塞性肺疾病，肺炎史。既往动脉血气、肺功能检查结果。

4. 家族史

哮喘，过敏，花粉症，特应性皮炎家族史。

5. 社会史

吸烟，酗酒。

6. 体格检查

一般表现：注意对患者病情的一般印象。呼吸困难，呼吸窘迫，出汗，嗜睡，焦虑，面色苍白。

Vital Signs: Temperature, respiratory rate (tachypnea >28 breaths/min), pulse (tachycardia), BP (widened pulse pressure, hypotension), pulsus paradoxus (inspiratory drop in systolic blood pressure >10 mmHg = severe attack).

HEENT: Nasal flaring, pharyngeal erythema, cyanosis, jugular venous distention.

Chest: Expiratory wheeze, rhonchi, decreased intensity of breath sounds (emphysema); sternocleidomastoid muscle contractions, barrel chest, increased anteroposterior diameter (hyperinflation); intracostal and supraclavicular retractions.

Heart: Decreased cardiac dullness to percussion (hyperinflation); distant heart sounds, third heart sound gallop (S3, cor pulmonale); increased intensity of pulmonic component of second heart sound (pulmonary hypertension).

Abdomen: Retractions, tenderness.

Extremities: Cyanosis, clubbing, edema.

Skin: Rash, urticaria.

Neuro: Decreased mental status, confusion.

7. Labs

Chest X-ray: hyperinflation, bullae, flattening of diaphragms; small, elongated heart.

ABG: Respiratory alkalosis, hypoxia.

Sputum gram stain; CBC, electrolytes, theophylline level.

ECG: Sinus tachycardia, right axis deviation, right ventricular hypertrophy. Pulmonary function tests, peak flow rate.

8. Differential Diagnosis

Asthma, bronchitis, COPD, pneumonia, congestive heart failure, anaphylaxis, upper airway obstruction, endobronchial tumors, carcinoid.

生命体征：体温，呼吸频率（呼吸急促> 28 bpm），脉搏（心动过速），血压（脉压增宽，低血压），反常脉搏（吸气时收缩压下降> 10 mmHg = 严重发作）。

头眼耳鼻喉：鼻翼扇动，咽部红斑，发绀，颈静脉怒张。

胸部：呼气性喘息，干啰音，呼吸音低（肺气肿）；胸锁乳突肌收缩，桶状胸，前后径增大（过度充气）；肋间隙和锁骨上窝凹陷。

心脏：心脏叩诊浊音减轻（过度充气），心音遥远，S3 奔马律（肺心病）；第二心音肺动脉瓣成分增强（肺动脉高压）。

腹部：凹陷，压痛。

肢体：发绀，杵状指，水肿。

皮肤：皮疹，荨麻疹。

神经系统：精神状态下降，意识模糊。

7. 实验室检查

胸片：过度充气，大疱，膈肌变平；心影细长。

动脉血气分析：呼吸性碱中毒，低氧血症。

痰革兰氏染色；血常规，电解质，茶碱水平。

心电图：窦性心动过速，右轴偏移，右心室肥大。肺功能检查，峰值流量。

8. 鉴别诊断

哮喘，支气管炎，慢性阻塞性肺疾病，肺炎，充血性心力衰竭，过敏反应，上呼吸道阻塞，支气管内肿瘤，类癌。

十、咯血（Hemoptysis）

1. Chief Complaint

The patient is a 78-year-old white male who has been coughing up blood for one day.

2. History of the Present Illness

Quantify the amount of blood, acuteness of onset, color (bright red, dark), character (coffee grounds, clots); dyspnea, chest pain (left or right), fever, chills; past bronchoscopies, exposure to tuberculosis; hematuria, weight loss, anorexia, hoarseness. Farm exposure, homelessness, residence in a nursing home, immigration from a foreign country. Smoking, leg pain or swelling (pulmonary embolism), bronchitis, aspiration of food or foreign body.

3. Past Medical History

COPD, heart failure, HIV risk factors (pulmonary Kaposi's sarcoma). Prior chest X-rays, CT scans, tuberculin testing (PPD).

4. Medications

Anticoagulants, aspirin, NSAIDs.

5. Family history

Bleeding disorders.

6. Physical Examination

General Appearance: Dyspnea, respiratory distress. Anxiety, diaphoresis, pallor.

Vital Signs: Temperature, respiratory rate (tachypnea), pulse (tachycardia), BP (hypotension); assess hemodynamic status.

Skin: Petechiae, ecchymoses (coagulopathy); cyanosis, purple plaques (Kaposi's sarcoma); rashes (paraneoplastic syndromes).

十、咯　血

1. 主　诉

78 岁的白人男性，咯血 1 天。

2. 现病史

咯血量，急性发病，颜色（红，黑），性状（咖啡渣，血块）；呼吸困难，胸痛（左右），发烧，寒战；既往支气管镜检查，肺结核接触史；血尿，体重下降，厌食，声音嘶哑。农场暴露，无家可归，养老院居住，国外移民。吸烟，腿痛或肿胀（肺栓塞），支气管炎，食物或异物误吸。

3. 既往史

慢性阻塞性肺疾病，心力衰竭，HIV 危险因素（肺卡波西氏肉瘤）。既往胸片，CT 扫描，结核菌素试验。

4. 药物史

抗凝剂，阿司匹林，非甾体抗炎药。

5. 家族史

出血性疾病。

6. 体格检查

一般情况：呼吸困难，呼吸窘迫。焦虑，发汗，面色苍白。

生命体征：体温，呼吸频率（呼吸急促），脉搏（心动过速），血压（低血压）；评估血流动力学状态。

皮肤：瘀点，瘀斑（凝血病），发绀，紫色斑块（卡波济肉瘤），皮疹（副肿瘤综合征）。

HEENT: Nasal or oropharyngeal lesions, tongue lacerations; telangiectasias on buccal mucosa (Rendu-Osler Weber disease); ulcerations of nasal septum (Wegener's granulomatosus), jugular venous distention, gingival disease (aspiration).

Lymph Nodes: Cervical, scalene or supraclavicular adenopathy (Virchow's nodes, intrathoracic malignancy).

Chest: Stridor, tenderness of chest wall; rhonchi, apical crackles (tuberculosis); localized wheezing (foreign body, malignancy), basilar crackles (pulmonary edema), pleural friction rub, breast masses (metastasis).

Heart: Mitral stenosis murmur (diastolic rumble), right ventricular gallop; accentuated second heart sound (pulmonary embolism).

Abdomen: Masses, liver nodules (metastases), tenderness.

Extremities: Calf tenderness, calf swelling (pulmonary embolism); clubbing (pulmonary disease), edema, bone pain (metastasis).

Rectal: Occult blood.

7. Labs

Sputum Gram stain, cytology, acid fast bacteria stain; CBC, platelets, ABG; pH of expectorated blood (alkaline = pulmonary; acidic = GI); UA (hematuria); INR/PTT, bleeding time; creatinine, sputum fungal culture; anti-glomerular basement membrane antibody, antinuclear antibody; PPD, cryptococcus antigen. ECG, chest X-ray, CT scan, bronchoscopy, ventilation/perfusion scan.

8. Differential Diagnosis

Infection: Bronchitis, pneumonia, lung abscess, tuberculosis, fungal infection, bronchiectasis, broncholithiasis.

Neoplasms: Bronchogenic carcinoma, metastatic cancer, Kaposi's sarcoma.

头眼耳鼻喉：鼻或口咽部病变，舌裂伤；颊黏膜毛细血管扩张；鼻中隔溃疡（韦格纳肉芽肿），颈静脉怒张，牙龈疾病（误吸）。

淋巴结：颈部，斜角肌或锁骨上淋巴结肿大（魏尔啸淋巴结，胸腔内恶性肿瘤）。

胸部：喘鸣，胸壁压痛；干啰音，肺尖啰音（结核）；局部喘鸣（异物，恶性肿瘤），肺底啰音（肺水肿），胸膜摩擦音，乳腺肿块（转移）。

心脏：二尖瓣狭窄杂音（舒张期隆隆样），右心室奔马律；第二心音增强（肺栓塞）。

腹部：肿块，肝结节（转移），压痛。

肢体：小腿压痛，小腿肿胀（肺栓塞）；杵状指（肺部疾病），水肿，骨痛（转移）。

直肠：隐血。

7. 实验室检查

痰革兰氏染色，细胞学，抗酸染色； 血常规，血小板，动脉血气分析；咯血 pH 值（碱性 = 肺；酸性 = 消化道）；尿常规（血尿）； 国际标准化比值/部分凝血活酶时间，出血时间；肌酐，痰真菌培养；抗肾小球基底膜抗体，抗核抗体； 结核菌素试验，隐球菌抗原。心电图，胸片，CT 扫描，支气管镜检查，通气/灌注扫描。

8. 鉴别诊断

感染：支气管炎，肺炎，肺脓肿，肺结核，真菌感染，支气管扩张，支气管结石症。

肿瘤：支气管癌，转移癌，卡波济肉瘤。

Vascular: Pulmonary embolism, mitral stenosis, pulmonary edema.

Miscellaneous: Trauma, foreign body, aspiration, coagulopathy, epistaxis, oropharyngeal bleeding, vasculitis, lupus, hemosiderosis, Wegener's granulomatosis.

血管：肺栓塞，二尖瓣狭窄，肺水肿。

其他：创伤，异物，误吸，凝血病，鼻出血，口咽出血，血管炎，系统性红斑狼疮，含铁血黄素沉着症，韦格纳肉芽肿。

十一、呕血（Hematemesis）

1. Chief Complaint

The patient is a 56-year-old white male with peptic ulcer disease who complains of emesis of blood for 2 hours.

2. History of the Present Illness

Duration and frequency of hematemesis (bright red blood, coffee ground material), volume of blood, hematocrit. Abdominal pain, melena, hematochezia (bright red blood per rectum); history of peptic ulcer, esophagitis, prior bleeding episodes. Nose bleeds, syncope, lightheadedness, nausea. Ingestion of alcohol. Weight loss, malaise, fatigue, anorexia, early satiety, jaundice. Nasogastric aspirate quantity and character; transfusions given previously.

3. Past Medical History

Liver or renal disease, hepatic encephalopathy, esophageal varices, aortic surgery. Past testing: X-ray studies, endoscopy. Past treatment: Endoscopic sclerotherapy, shunt surgery.

4. Medications

Aspirin, nonsteroidal anti-inflammatory drugs, steroids, anticoagulants.

5. Family History

Liver disease or bleeding disorders.

6. Physical Examination

General Appearance: Pallor, diaphoresis, cold extremities, confusion.

Vital Signs: Supine and upright pulse and blood pressure (orthostatic hypotension; resting tachycardia indicates a 10% blood volume loss; postural hypotension indicates a 20%-30% blood loss); oliguria (<20 mL of urine per hour), temperature.

十一、呕　血

1. 主　诉

56 岁白人男性，消化性溃疡患者，呕血 2 小时。

2. 现病史

呕血的持续时间和频率（鲜红色血，咖啡渣样），呕血量，血细胞比容。腹痛，黑便，便血（直肠出血为鲜红色）；消化性溃疡，食管炎史，既往出血史。鼻衄，晕厥，头晕，恶心，饮酒，体重减轻，全身乏力，疲劳，厌食，早饱，黄疸，胃抽吸物的量和特征；既往输血史。

3. 既往史

肝肾疾病，肝性脑病，食管静脉曲张，主动脉手术。既往检查：X 射线检查，内窥镜检查。既往治疗：内窥镜硬化疗法，分流手术。

4. 药物史

阿司匹林，非甾体消炎药，类固醇，抗凝剂。

5. 家族史

肝病或出血性疾病。

6. 体格检查

一般情况：面色苍白，发汗，四肢发冷，精神错乱。

生命体征：卧位和直立位脉搏和血压（直立性低血压；静息性心动过速示血容量减少 10%；直立性低血压示血流量减少 20% ~ 30%）；少尿（每小时尿量<20 mL），体位。

Skin: Delayed capillary refill, pallor, petechiae. Stigmata of liver disease (jaundice, umbilical venous collaterals [caput medusae], spider angiomas, parotid gland hypertrophy). Hemorrhagic telangiectasia (Osler-Weber-Rendu syndrome), abnormal pigmentation (Peutz-Jeghers syndrome); purple-brown nodules (Kaposi's sarcoma).

HEENT: Scleral pallor, oral telangiectasia, flat neck veins.

Chest: Gynecomastia (cirrhosis), breast masses (metastatic disease).

Heart: Systolic ejection murmur.

Abdomen: Scars, tenderness, rebound, masses, splenomegaly, hepatic atrophy (cirrhosis), liver nodules. Ascites, dilated abdominal veins.

Extremities: Dupuytren's contracture (palmar contractures, cirrhosis), edema.

Neuro: Decreased mental status, confusion, poor memory, asterixis (hepatic encephalopathy).

Genitourinary/Rectal: Gross or occult blood, masses, testicular atrophy.

7. Labs

CBC, platelets, electrolytes, BUN (elevation suggests upper GI bleed), glucose, INR/PTT, ECG. Endoscopy, nuclear scan, angiography.

8. Differential Diagnosis of Upper GI Bleeding

Gastric or duodenal ulcer, esophageal varices, Mallory Weiss tear (gastroesophageal junction tear due to vomiting or retching), gastritis, esophagitis, swallowed blood (nose bleed, oral lesion), duodenitis, gastric cancer, vascular ectasias, coagulopathy, aorto-enteric fistula.

皮肤：毛细血管充盈延迟，面色苍白，瘀斑。肝病体征﹝黄疸，脐周静脉曲张（海蛇头），蜘蛛痣，腮腺肥大﹞。出血性毛细血管扩张（Osler-Weber-Rendu 综合征），色素异常沉着（Peutz-Jeghers 综合征）；紫褐色结节（卡波西氏肉瘤）。

头眼耳鼻喉：巩膜苍白，口腔毛细血管扩张，颈静脉扁平。

胸部：男性乳房发育（肝硬化），乳房包块（转移性疾病）。

心脏：收缩期喷射性杂音。

腹部：疤痕，压痛，肌卫，肿块，脾大，肝萎缩（肝硬化），肝结节。腹水，腹部静脉扩张。

肢体：Dupuytren 氏挛缩（掌挛缩，肝硬化），水肿。

神经系统：精神状态下降，意识模糊，记忆力差，扑翼样震颤（肝性脑病）。

泌尿生殖系统/直肠：肉眼可见血或隐血，肿块，睾丸萎缩。

7. 实验室检查

血常规，血小板，电解质，尿素氮（升高提示上消化道出血），葡萄糖，国际标准化比值/部分凝血活酶时间，心电图。内窥镜检查，核素扫描，血管造影。

8. 上消化道出血鉴别诊断

胃或十二指肠溃疡，食管静脉曲张，马洛韦斯氏撕裂（剧烈呕吐引起的胃食管连接处撕裂），胃炎，食管炎，吞血（鼻出血，口腔病变），十二指肠炎，胃癌，血管扩张症，凝血病，主动脉肠瘘。

十二、便血（Melena）

1. Chief Complaint

The patient is a 75-year-old male with diverticulosis who complains of rectal bleeding for 8 hours.

2. History of the Present Illness

Duration, quantity, color of bleeding (gross blood, streaks on stool, melena), recent hematocrit. Change in bowel habits or stool caliber, abdominal pain, fever. Constipation, diarrhea, anorectal pain. Epistaxis, anorexia, weight loss, malaise, vomiting. Color of nasogastric aspirate. Fecal mucus, tenesmus, lightheadedness.

3. Past Medical History

Diverticulosis, hemorrhoids, colitis, peptic ulcer, hematemesis, bleeding disease, coronary or renal disease, cirrhosis, alcoholism, easy bruising.

Past Testing: Barium enema, colonoscopy, sigmoidoscopy, upper GI series.

4. Medications

Anticoagulants, aspirin, NSAIDS.

5. Physical Examination

General Appearance: Signs of dehydration, pallor.

Vital Signs: BP, pulse (orthostatic hypotension), respiratory rate, temperature (tachycardia), oliguria.

Skin: Cold, clammy skin; delayed capillary refill, pallor, jaundice. Stigmata of liver disease: Umbilical venous collaterals (Caput medusae), jaundice, spider angiomata, parotid gland hypertrophy, gynecomastia. Rashes, purpura, buccal mucosa discolorations or pigmentation.

HEENT: Atherosclerotic retinal disease, "silver wire" arteries .

Heart: Systolic ejection murmurs, atrial fibrillation (mesenteric emboli).

十二、便　血

1. 主　诉

75 岁男性，憩室病患者直肠出血 8 小时。

2. 现病史

出血持续时间，量，颜色（肉眼可见血，大便带血，黑便），近期血细胞比容。排便习惯改变或大便性状，腹痛，发热，便秘，腹泻，肛门直肠痛。鼻衄，厌食，体重减轻，全身乏力，呕吐。胃抽吸物的颜色，黏液便，里急后重，头晕。

3. 既往史

憩室病，痔疮，结肠炎，消化性溃疡，呕血，出血病，冠状动脉或肾脏疾病，肝硬化，酒精中毒，易瘀伤。

既往检查：钡餐，结肠镜检查，乙状结肠镜检查，上消化道检查系列。

4. 药物史

抗凝剂，阿司匹林，非甾体抗炎药。

5. 体格检查

一般情况：脱水迹象，面色苍白。

生命体征：血压，脉搏（直立性低血压），呼吸频率，体温（心动过速），少尿。

皮肤：寒冷，湿润的皮肤；毛细血管充盈延迟，面色苍白，黄疸。肝病体征：脐周静脉曲张（海蛇头），黄疸，蜘蛛痣，腮腺肥大，男性乳房发育症。皮疹，紫癜，颊黏膜变色或色素沉着。

头眼耳鼻喉：动脉粥样硬化性视网膜疾病，"银丝"动脉。

心脏：收缩期喷射性杂音，房颤（肠系膜动脉栓塞）。

Abdomen: Scars, bruits, masses, distention, rebound tenderness, hernias, liver atrophy (cirrhosis), splenomegaly. Ascites, pulsatile masses (aortic aneurysm).

Genitourinary: Testicular atrophy.

Extremities: Cold, pale extremities.

Neuro: Decreased mental status, confusion, asterixis (hepatic encephalopathy).

Rectal: Gross or occult blood, masses, hemorrhoids; fissures, polyps, ulcers.

6. Labs

CBC (anemia), liver function tests, ammonia level. Abdominal X-ray series (thumbprinting, air fluid levels).

7. Differential Diagnosis of Lower Gastrointestinal Bleeding

Hemorrhoids, fissures, diverticulosis, upper GI bleeding, rectal trauma, inflammatory bowel disease, infectious colitis, ischemic colitis, bleeding polyps, carcinoma, angiodysplasias, intussusception, coagulopathies, Meckel's diverticulitis, endometriosis, aortoenteric fistula.

腹部：疤痕，杂音，肿块，扩张，反跳痛，疝气，肝萎缩（肝硬化），脾肿大，腹水，搏动性肿块（主动脉瘤）。

泌尿生殖道：睾丸萎缩。

四肢：寒冷苍白的四肢。

神经系统：精神状态下降，意识模糊，扑翼样震颤（肝性脑病）。

直肠：肉眼可见出血或隐血，肿块，痔疮；肛裂，息肉，溃疡。

6. 实验室检查

血常规（贫血），肝功能，血氨水平。腹部 X 射线系列（指印征，气液平）。

7. 下消化道出血鉴别诊断

痔疮，肛裂，憩室病，上消化道出血，直肠外伤，炎症性肠病，感染性结肠炎，缺血性结肠炎，息肉出血，癌，血管发育异常，肠套叠，凝血病，梅克尔憩室炎，子宫内膜异位症，主动脉肠瘘。

十三、血尿（Hematuria）

1. Chief Complaint

The patient is a 65-year-old male who complains of bloody urine for 4 days.

2. History of the Present Illness

Quantity of RBCs found on urinalysis. Repeat testing. Color, timing, pattern of hematuria: Initial hematuria (anterior urethral lesion); terminal hematuria (bladder neck or prostate lesion); hematuria throughout voiding (bladder or upper urinary tract). Frequency, dysuria, suprapubic pain, flank pain (renal colic), perineal pain; fever. Recent exercise, menstruation; bleeding between voidings. Foley catheterization, joint pain. Recent sore throat, streptococcal skin infection (glomerulonephritis).

3. Past Medical History

Prior pyelonephritis; occupational exposure to toxins.

4. Medications Associated with Hematuria

Warfarin, aspirin, ibuprofen, naproxen, phenobarbital, allopurinol, phenytoin, cyclophosphamide.

5. Causes of Red Urine

Pyridium, phenytoin, ibuprofen, cascara laxatives, levodopa, methyldopa, quinine, rifampin, berries, fava beans, food coloring, rhubarb, beets, hemoglobinuria, myoglobinuria.

6. Family History

Hematuria, renal disease, sickle cell, bleeding diathesis, deafness (Alport's syndrome), hypertension.

7. Physical Examination

General Appearance: Signs of dehydration.

Vital Signs: BP (hypertension), pulse (tachycardia), respiratory rate, temperature (fever).

十三、血　尿

1. 主　诉

65 岁白人男性，血尿 4 天。

2. 现病史

尿分析中红细胞数量。重复检测。血尿的颜色，时间，模式：初始血尿（尿道前部病变）；终末血尿（膀胱颈或前列腺病变）；全程血尿（膀胱或上尿路）。排尿频率，排尿困难，耻骨上区痛，胁腹痛（肾绞痛），会阴痛；发热。近期运动，月经；排尿间隙出血。导尿管，关节痛，近期喉咙痛，皮肤链球菌感染（肾小球肾炎）。

3. 既往史

既往肾盂肾炎；职业性毒物暴露。

4. 血尿相关的药物

华法林，阿司匹林，布洛芬，萘普生，苯巴比妥，别嘌醇，苯妥英钠，环磷酰胺。

5. 致尿液变红的因素

吡啶鎓，苯妥英钠，布洛芬，卡斯卡拉泻药，左旋多巴，甲基多巴，奎宁，利福平，浆果，蚕豆，食用色素，大黄，甜菜，血红蛋白尿，肌红蛋白尿。

6. 家族史

血尿，肾脏疾病，镰状细胞，出血性疾病，耳聋（阿尔波特综合征），高血压。

7. 体格检查

一般情况：脱水迹象。

生命体征：血压（高血压），脉搏（心动过速），呼吸频率，体温（发热）。

207

Skin: Rashes.

HEENT: Pharyngitis, carotid bruits.

Heart: Heart murmur; irregular rhythm (atrial fibrillation, renal emboli).

Abdomen: Tenderness, masses, costovertebral angle tenderness (renal calculus or pyelonephritis), abdominal bruits, nephromegaly, suprapubic tenderness.

Genitourinary: Urethral lesions, discharge, condyloma, foreign body, cervical malignancy; prostate tenderness, nodules, or enlargement (prostatitis, prostate cancer).

Extremities: Peripheral edema (nephrotic syndrome), arthritis, ecchymoses, petechiae, unequal peripheral pulses (aortic dissection).

8. Labs

CBC, KUB, intravenous pyelogram, ultrasound. Streptozyme panel, INR/PTT.

Indicators of Significant Hematuria: ①>3 RBC's per high-power field on 2 of 3 specimens; ②>100 RBC's per HPF in 1 specimen; ③ gross hematuria The patient should abstain from exercise for 48 hours prior to urine collection, and urine should not be collected during menses.

9. Differential Diagnosis

(1) Medical Hematuria is caused by a glomerular lesion; plasma proteins filter into urine out of proportion to the amount of hematuria. It is characterized by glomerular RBCs that are distorted with crenated membranes and an uneven hemoglobin distribution and casts. Microscopic hematuria and a urine dipstick test of 2+ protein is more likely to have a medical cause.

皮肤：皮疹。

头眼耳鼻喉：咽炎，颈动脉杂音。

心脏：心脏杂音；节律不规则（房颤，肾栓塞）。

腹部：压痛，肿块，肋脊角压痛（肾结石或肾盂肾炎），腹部杂音，肾肿大，耻骨上区压痛。

泌尿生殖系统：尿道病变，分泌物，尖锐湿疣，异物，宫颈恶性肿瘤；前列腺压痛，结节或肿大（前列腺炎，前列腺癌）。

肢体：外周水肿（肾病综合征），关节炎，瘀点，瘀斑，外周脉搏不对等（主动脉夹层）。

8. 实验室检查

血常规，泌尿系（肾脏输尿管膀胱）摄片，静脉肾盂造影，超声检查，链球菌酶，国际标准化比值/部分凝血活酶时间。

有意义血尿的指标：① 送检 2 ~ 3 次样本中每高倍视野中>3 个红细胞；② 单次送检样本每高倍视野中>100 个红细胞；③ 肉眼血尿，收集尿液前 48 小时不运动且避开月经期。

9. 鉴别诊断

（1）肾小球病变所致血尿：血浆蛋白会与血尿量不成比例的过滤到尿液中。特征是红细胞经肾小球被锯齿状膜扭曲，血红蛋白分布不均匀、有管型。镜下血尿和尿液试纸检测 2+蛋白提示该原因所致。

(2) Urologic Hematuria is caused by a urologic lesion, such as a urinary stone or carcinoma; it is characterized by minimal proteinuria, and protein appears in urine proportional to the amount of whole blood present. RBCs are disk shaped with an even hemoglobin distribution; there is an absence of casts.

（2）泌尿系统其他病变：如泌尿系结石或癌；特点是蛋白尿极少，尿液中蛋白质的含量与全血中的含量成比例。红细胞呈圆盘状，血红蛋白分布均匀，无管型。

十四、恶心&呕吐（Nausea & Vomiting）

1. Chief Complaint

The patient is a 62-year-old female with diabetes who complains of vomiting for 4 hours.

2. History of the Present Illness

Character of emesis (color, food, bilious, feculent, hematemesis, coffee ground material, projectile); abdominal pain, effect of vomiting on pain; early satiety, fever, melena, vertigo, tinnitus (labyrinthitis). Clay colored stools, dark urine, jaundice (biliary obstruction); recent change in medications. Ingestion of spoiled food; exposure to ill contacts; dysphagia, odynophagia. Possibility of pregnancy (last menstrual period, contraception, sexual history).

3. Past Medical History

Diabetes, cardiac disease, peptic ulcer, liver disease, CNS disease, headache. X-rays, upper GI series, endoscopy.

4. Medications Associated with Nausea

Digoxin, colchicine, theophylline, chemotherapy, anticholinergics, morphine, meperidine, oral contraceptives, progesterone, antiarrhythmics, erythromycin, antibiotics, antidepressants.

5. Physical Examination

General Appearance: Signs of dehydration, septic appearance.

Vital Signs: BP (orthostatic hypotension), pulse (tachycardia), respiratory rate, temperature (fever).

Skin: Pallor, jaundice, spider angiomas.

HEENT: Nystagmus, papilledema; ketone odor on breath (apple odor, diabetic ketoacidosis); jugular venous distention or flat neck veins.

Abdomen: Scars, bowel sounds, bruits, tenderness, rebound, rigidity, distention, hepatomegaly, ascites.

十四、恶心＆呕吐

1. 主　诉

62 岁女性糖尿病患者，呕吐 4 小时。

2. 现病史

呕吐的特征（颜色，食物，胆汁，残渣，呕血，咖啡渣，喷射样）；腹痛，呕吐对疼痛的影响；早饱，发烧，黑便，眩晕，耳鸣（迷路炎）。黏土色的粪便，深色尿液，黄疸（胆管阻塞）；近期药物变化。摄入变质的食物；疾病接触史；吞咽困难，吞咽痛。怀孕的可能性（末次月经，避孕，性生活史）。

3. 既往史

糖尿病，心脏病，消化性溃疡，肝病，中枢神经系统疾病，头痛。X 射线，上消化道检查系列，内窥镜检查。

4. 恶心相关的药物

地高辛，秋水仙碱，茶碱，化疗，抗胆碱能药，吗啡，哌替啶，口服避孕药，黄体酮，抗心律失常药，红霉素，抗生素，抗抑郁药。

5. 体格检查

一般情况：脱水迹象，败血症外观。

生命体征：血压（直立性低血压），脉搏（心动过速），呼吸频率，体温（发热）。

皮肤：苍白，黄疸，蜘蛛痣。

头眼耳鼻喉：眼球震颤，视乳头水肿；呼气酮味（苹果味，糖尿病性酮症酸中毒），颈静脉怒张或颈静脉扁平。

腹部：疤痕，肠鸣音，杂音，压痛，肌卫，僵硬，扩张，肝肿大，腹水。

Extremities: Edema, cyanosis.

Rectal: Masses, occult blood.

6. Labs

CBC, electrolytes, UA, amylase, lipase, LFTs, pregnancy test, abdominal X-ray series.

7. Differential Diagnosis

Gastroenteritis, systemic infections, medications (contraceptives, antiarrhythmics, chemotherapy, antibiotics), pregnancy, appendicitis, peptic ulcer, cholecystitis, hepatitis, intestinal obstruction, gastroesophageal reflux, gastroparesis, ileus, pancreatitis, myocardial ischemia, tumors (esophageal, gastric), increased intracranial pressure, labyrinthitis, diabetic ketoacidosis, renal failure, toxins, bulimia, psychogenic vomiting.

四肢：水肿，发绀。

直肠：肿块，隐血。

6. 实验室检查

血常规，电解质，尿常规，淀粉酶，脂肪酶，肝功能，妊娠试验，腹部摄片。

7. 鉴别诊断

胃肠炎，全身感染，药物（避孕药，抗心律失常药，化疗药，抗生素），怀孕，阑尾炎，消化性溃疡，胆囊炎，肝炎，肠梗阻，胃食管反流，胃轻瘫，肠梗阻，胰腺炎，心肌缺血，肿瘤（食管，胃），颅内压增高，迷路炎，糖尿病酮症酸中毒，肾衰，毒素，贪食症，精神性呕吐。

十五、厌食&体重下降（Anorexia & Weight Loss）

1. Chief Complaint

The patient is a 63-year-old male with diabetes who complains of loss of appetite and weight loss for one week.

2. History of the Present Illness

Time of onset, amount and rate of weight loss (suddenly, gradually); change in appetite, nausea, vomiting, dysphagia, abdominal pain; exacerbation of pain with eating (intestinal angina); diarrhea, fever, chills, night sweats; dental problems; restricted access to food. Polyuria, polydipsia; skin or hair changes; dyspepsia, jaundice, dysuria; cough, change in bowel habits; chronic illness. Dietary restrictions (low salt, low fat); diminished taste, malignancy, AIDS risks factors; psychiatric disease, renal disease, alcoholism, drug abuse (cocaine, amphetamines).

3. Physical Examination

General Appearance: Muscle wasting, cachexia.

Vital Signs: Pulse (bradycardia), BP, respiratory rate, temperature (hypothermia).

Skin: Pallor, jaundice, hair changes, skin laxity, cheilosis, dermatitis (Pellagra).

HEENT: Dental erosions induced vomiting, oropharyngeal lesions, thyromegaly, glossitis, temporal wasting, supraclavicular adenopathy (Virchow's node).

Chest: Rhonchi, barrel shaped chest.

Heart: Murmurs, displaced PMI.

Abdomen: Scars, decreased bowel sounds, tenderness, hepatomegaly splenomegaly. Periumbilical adenopathy, palpable masses.

十五、厌食＆体重下降

1. 主　诉

63 岁男性糖尿病患者，食欲不振和体重下降 1 周。

2. 现病史

起病时间，体重下降的量和速度（突然，逐渐）；食欲改变，恶心，呕吐，吞咽困难，腹痛；进食加剧疼痛（肠绞痛）；腹泻，发热，寒战，盗汗；牙齿问题；食物不足。多尿，多饮；皮肤或头发的变化；消化不良，黄疸，排尿困难；咳嗽，排便习惯改变；慢性病。饮食限制（低盐低脂）；味觉下降，恶性肿瘤，艾滋病危险因素；精神疾病，肾脏疾病，酒精中毒，药物滥用（可卡因，苯丙胺）。

3. 体格检查

一般表现：肌肉萎缩，恶病质。

生命体征：脉搏（心动过缓），血压，呼吸频率，体温（体温过低）。

皮肤：面色苍白，黄疸，毛发变化，皮肤松弛，口角干裂，皮炎。

头眼耳鼻喉：齿病所致呕吐，口咽部病变，甲状腺肿大，舌炎，颞部消瘦，锁骨上淋巴结肿大（魏尔啸淋巴结）。

胸部：干啰音，桶状胸。

心脏：杂音，最强心尖搏动点移位。

腹部：疤痕，肠鸣音减弱，压痛，肝肿大，脾肿大。脐周腺病，可触及肿块。

Extremities: Edema, muscle wasting, lymphadenopathy, skin abrasions on fingers.

Neurologic: Decreased sensation, poor proprioception.

Rectal: Occult blood, masses.

4. Labs

CBC, electrolytes, albumin, pre-albumin, transferrin, thyroid studies, LFTs, toxicology screen.

5. Differential Diagnosis

Inadequate caloric intake, peptic ulcer, depression, anorexia nervosa, dementia, hyper/hypothyroidism, cardiopulmonary disease, narcotics, diminished taste, diminished olfaction, poor dental hygiene (loose dentures), cholelithiasis, malignancy (gastric carcinoma), gastritis, hepatic or renal failure, infection, alcohol abuse, AIDS.

四肢：水肿，肌肉萎缩，淋巴结肿大，手指上的皮肤擦伤。

神经系统：感觉减退，本体感觉差。

直肠：隐血，肿块。

4. 实验室检查

血常规，电解质，白蛋白，前白蛋白，转铁蛋白，甲状腺功能，肝功能，毒物学筛查。

5. 鉴别诊断

热量摄入不足，消化性溃疡，抑郁症，神经性厌食症，痴呆，甲状腺功能亢进/甲状腺功能减退，心肺疾病，麻醉药，味觉下降，嗅觉下降，牙齿卫生差（假牙松动），胆石症，恶性肿瘤（胃癌），胃炎，肝肾衰，感染，酗酒，艾滋病。

十六、腹泻（Diarrhea）

1. Chief Complaint

The patient is a 52-year-old white male who complains of diarrhea for two days.

2. History of the Present Illness

Rate of onset, duration, frequency. Volume of stool output (number of stools per day), watery stools; fever. Abdominal cramps, bloating, flatulence, tenesmus, anorexia, nausea, vomiting, bloating; myalgias, arthralgias, weight loss. Stool Appearance: Buoyancy, blood or mucus, oily, foul odor. Recent ingestion of spoiled poultry (salmonella), milk, seafood (shrimp, shellfish; Vibrio parahaemolyticus); restaurants, travel history, laxative abuse. Ill contacts with diarrhea, inflammatory bowel disease; family history of celiac disease.

3. Past Medical History

Sexual exposures, immunosuppressive agents, AIDS risk factors, coronary artery disease, peripheral vascular disease (ischemic colitis). Exacerbation by stress.

4. Medications Associated with Diarrhea

Laxatives, magnesium-containing antacids, sulfa drugs, antibiotics (erythromycin, clindamycin), cholinergic agents, colchicine, milk (lactase deficiency), gum (sorbitol).

5. Physical Examination

General Appearance: Signs of dehydration or malnutrition. Septic appearance.

Vital Signs: BP (orthostatic hypotension), pulse (tachycardia), respiratory rate, temperature (fever).

Skin: Decreased skin turgor, skin mottling, delayed capillary refill, jaundice.

十六、腹　泻

1. 主　诉

52 岁白人男性，腹泻 2 天。

2. 现病史

起病速度，持续时间，频率。粪便量（每日解便次数），水样便；发热。腹部绞痛，腹胀，胃肠胀气，里急后重，厌食，恶心，呕吐，腹胀；肌痛，关节痛，体重减轻。大便外观：漂浮，血性或黏液，油性，难闻的气味。近期摄入变质的家禽（沙门氏菌），牛奶，海鲜（虾，贝类；副溶血弧菌），餐馆，旅行史，泻药滥用。腹泻，炎性肠病接触史；乳糜泻家族史。

3. 既往史

性接触，免疫抑制剂，艾滋病危险因素，冠状动脉疾病，周围血管疾病（缺血性结肠炎）。压力加剧。

4. 腹泻有关的药物

泻药，含镁的抗酸剂，磺胺药，抗生素（红霉素，克林霉素），胆碱能药，秋水仙碱，牛奶（乳糖酶缺乏症），口香糖（山梨糖醇）。

5. 体格检查

一般情况：脱水或营养不良的迹象。败血症的外观。

生命体征：血压（直立性低血压），脉搏（心动过速），呼吸频率，体温（发热）。

皮肤：皮肤弹性下降，皮肤斑点，毛细血管充盈延迟，黄疸。

HEENT: Oral ulcers (inflammatory bowel disease), dry mucous membranes, cheilosis (cracked lips, riboflavin deficiency); glossitis (B_{12}, folate deficiency). Oropharyngeal candidiasis (AIDS).

Abdomen: Hyperactive bowel sounds, tenderness, rebound, guarding, rigidity (peritonitis), distention, hepatomegaly, bruits (ischemic colitis).

Extremities: Arthritis (ulcerative colitis). Absent peripheral pulses, bruits (ischemic colitis).

Rectal: Perianal ulcers, sphincter tone, tenderness, masses, occult blood.

Neuro: Mental status changes. Peripheral neuropathy (B_6, B_{12} deficiency), decreased perianal sensation, sphincter reflex.

6. Labs

Electrolytes, Wright's stain for fecal leukocytes; cultures for enteric pathogens, ova and parasites × 3; clostridium difficile toxin. CBC with differential, albumin, flexible sigmoidoscopy.

Abdominal X-ray: Air fluid levels, dilation, pancreatic calcifications.

7. Differential Diagnosis

Acute Infectious Diarrhea: Infectious diarrhea (salmonella, shigella, E coli, Campylobacter, Bacillus cereus), enteric viruses (rotavirus, Norwalk virus), traveler's diarrhea, antibiotic-related diarrhea

Chronic Diarrhea

Osmotic Diarrhea: Laxatives, lactulose, lactase deficiency (gastroenteritis, sprue), other disaccharidase deficiencies, ingestion of mannitol, sorbitol, enteral feeding.

Secretory Diarrhea: Bacterial enterotoxins, viral infection; AIDS-associated disorders (mycobacterial, HIV enteropathy), Zollinger-Ellison syndrome, vasoactive intestinal peptide tumor, carcinoid tumors, medullary thyroid cancer, colonic villus adenoma.

头眼耳鼻喉：口腔溃疡（炎性肠病），黏膜干燥，口唇炎（嘴唇开裂，核黄素缺乏）；舌炎（维生素 B_{12}，叶酸缺乏）。口咽念珠菌病（艾滋病）。

腹部：肠蠕动亢进，压痛，反跳痛，肌卫，僵硬（腹膜炎），扩张，肝肿大，杂音（缺血性结肠炎）。

肢体：关节炎（溃疡性结肠炎）。外周脉搏消失，杂音（缺血性结肠炎）。

直肠：肛周溃疡，括约肌张力，压痛，肿块，隐血。

神经系统：精神状态改变。周围神经病变（维生素 B_6，B_{12} 缺乏），肛周感觉、括约肌反射下降。

6. 实验室检查

电解质，粪便白细胞的赖特氏染色；肠道病原体，卵和寄生虫的培养物 ×3；艰难梭菌毒素。血常规及分类，白蛋白，乙状结肠镜检查。

腹部 X 片：气液平，扩张，胰腺钙化。

7. 鉴别诊断

急性感染性腹泻：感染性腹泻（沙门氏菌，志贺氏菌，大肠杆菌，弯曲杆菌，蜡状芽孢杆菌），肠病毒（轮状病毒，诺沃克病毒），旅行者腹泻，抗生素相关性腹泻

慢性腹泻

渗透性腹泻：泻药，乳果糖，乳糖酶缺乏症（胃肠炎，口炎性腹泻），其他双糖酶缺乏症，服用甘露醇、山梨醇，肠内喂养。

分泌性腹泻：细菌肠毒素，病毒感染；艾滋病相关疾病（分枝杆菌，HIV 肠病），佐林格-埃里森综合征，血管活性肠肽肿瘤，类癌，甲状腺髓样癌，结肠绒毛腺瘤。

Exudative Diarrhea: Bacterial infection, Clostridium difficile, parasites, Crohn's disease, ulcerative colitis, diverticulitis, intestinal ischemia, diverticulitis.

Diarrhea Secondary to Altered Intestinal Motility: Diabetic gastroparesis, hyperthyroidism, laxatives, cholinergics, irritable bowel syndrome, bacterial overgrowth, constipation-related diarrhea.

渗出性腹泻：细菌感染，艰难梭菌，寄生虫，克罗恩病，溃疡性结肠炎，憩室炎，肠缺血，憩室炎。

肠动力相关性腹泻：糖尿病性胃轻瘫，甲状腺功能亢进，泻药，胆碱能药，肠易激综合征，细菌过度生长，便秘相关性腹泻。

十七、水肿 (Edema)

1. Chief Complaint

The patient is a 58-year-old male with hypertension who complains of ankle swelling for 2 days.

2. History of the Present Illness

Duration of edema; localized or generalized; leg pain, redness. History of heart failure, liver, or renal disease; weight gain, shortness of breath, malnutrition, chronic diarrhea (protein losing enteropathy), allergies, alcoholism. Exacerbation by upright position. Recent fluid input and output balance.

3. Past Medical History

Cardiac testing, chest X-rays. History of deep vein thrombosis, venous insufficiency.

4. Medications

Cardiac drugs, diuretics, calcium channel blockers.

5. Physical Examination

General Appearance: Respiratory distress, dyspnea, pallor, diaphoresis.

Vitals: BP (hypotension), pulse, temperature, respiratory rate.

HEENT: jugular venous distention at 45°; carotid pulse amplitude.

Chest: Breath sounds, crackles, wheeze, dullness to percussion.

Heart: Displacement of point of maximal impulse, atrial fibrillation (irregular rhythm); S3 gallop (LV dilation), friction rubs.

Abdomen: Abdominojugular reflux, ascites, hepatomegaly, splenomegaly, distention, fluid wave, shifting dullness, generalized tenderness.

十七、水　肿

1. 主　诉

58 岁男性，高血压，踝关节持续肿胀 2 天。

2. 现病史

水肿持续时间；局部或全身性；腿痛，发红。心力衰竭，肝脏或肾脏病病史；体重增加，呼吸困难，营养不良，慢性腹泻（蛋白质丢失性肠病），过敏，酗酒。直立姿势加剧。近期液体出入量平衡。

3. 既往史

心脏检查，胸片。深静脉血栓史，静脉功能不全史。

4. 药物史

心脏药物，利尿剂，钙通道阻滞剂。

5. 体格检查

一般情况：呼吸窘迫，呼吸困难，面色苍白，出汗。

生命体征：血压（低血压），脉搏，体温，呼吸频率。

头眼耳鼻喉：上半身 45°颈静脉怒张；颈动脉搏动幅度。

胸部：呼吸音、湿啰音，喘息音，叩诊浊音。

心脏：最强心尖搏动点移位，房颤（心律不齐）；S3 心音（左心室扩张），摩擦音。

腹部：腹颈静脉反流征，腹水，肝肿大，脾肿大，扩张，液波震颤，移动性浊音，全腹压痛。

Extremities: Pitting or non-pitting edema (graded 1 to 4+), redness, warmth; mottled brown discoloration of ankle skin (venous insufficiency); leg circumference, calf tenderness, Homan's sign (dorsiflexion elicits pain; thrombosis); pulses, cyanosis, clubbing.

Neurologic: Altered mental status.

6. Labs

Electrolytes, liver function tests, CBC, chest X-ray, ECG, cardiac enzymes, Doppler studies of lower extremities.

7. Differential Diagnosis of Edema

Generalized Edema: Heart failure, cirrhosis, acute glomerulonephritis, nephrotic syndrome, renal failure, obstruction of hepatic venous outflow, obstruction of inferior or superior vena cava.

Unilateral Edema: Deep venous thrombosis; lymphatic obstruction by tumor.

Endocrine: Mineralocorticoid excess, hypoalbuminemia.

Miscellaneous: Anemia, angioedema, iatrogenic edema.

肢体：凹陷性/非凹陷性水肿（1 至 4+级），发红，温暖；脚踝皮肤呈斑驳褐色（静脉功能不全）；腿围，小腿压痛，霍曼征（背屈引起疼痛；血栓形成）；脉搏，发绀，杵状指。

神经系统：精神状态改变。

6. 实验室检查

电解质，肝功能检查，血常规，胸片，心电图，心肌酶，下肢多普超声检查。

7. 水肿鉴别诊断

全身性水肿：心力衰竭，肝硬化，急性肾小球肾炎，肾病综合征，肾衰竭，肝静脉流出道阻塞，下腔静脉或上腔静脉阻塞。

单侧水肿：深静脉血栓形成；肿瘤所致淋巴阻塞。

内分泌性水肿：盐皮质激素过多，低白蛋白血症。

其他：贫血，血管性水肿，医源性水肿。

十八、少尿（Oliguria）

1. Chief Complaint

The patient is a 80-year-old female with diabetes who presents with decreased urine output for 8 hours.

2. History of the Present Illness

Oliguria (urine: <20 mL/h, 400-500 mL/d); anuria (urine: <100 mL/d); hemorrhage, heart failure, sepsis, vomiting, diarrhea, fever, chills; measured fluid input and output by Foley catheter; prostate enlargement, kidney stones, dysuria, flank pain. Abdominal pain, hematuria, passing of tissue fragments, foamy urine (proteinuria).

3. Past Medical History

Recent upper respiratory infection (post streptococcal glomerulonephritis), recent chemotherapy (tumor lysis syndrome).

4. Medications

Anticholinergics, nephrotoxic drugs (aminoglycosides, amphotericin, NSAID's), renally excreted medications.

5. Physical Examination

General Appearance: Signs of dehydration, septic appearance.

Vital Signs: BP; pulse (tachycardia); temperature (fever), respiratory rate (tachypnea).

Skin: Decreased skin turgor over sternum (hypovolemia); skin temperature and color; delayed capillary refill; jaundice (hepatorenal syndrome).

HEENT: Oral mucosa moisture, ocular moisture, flat neck veins (volume depletion), venous distention (heart failure).

Chest: Crackles (heart failure).

十八、少　尿

1. 主　诉

80 岁的女性，糖尿病患者，少尿 8 小时。

2. 现病史

少尿（尿液：<20 mL/h，400～500 mL/d）；无尿（尿液：<100 mL/d）；出血，心力衰竭，败血症，呕吐，腹泻，发热，寒战；置尿管监测尿量；前列腺肿大，肾结石，排尿困难，胁腹疼痛。腹痛，血尿，尿中含组织碎片，泡沫尿（蛋白尿）。

3. 既往史

近期上呼吸道感染（链球菌感染后肾小球肾炎），近期化疗（肿瘤溶解综合征）。

4. 药物史

抗胆碱药，肾毒性药物（氨基糖苷类，两性霉素，非甾体抗炎药），经肾脏排泄的药物。

5. 体格检查

一般情况：脱水迹象，败血症外观。

生命体征：血压；脉搏（心动过速）；温度（发热），呼吸频率（呼吸急促）。

皮肤：胸骨处皮肤弹性下降（血容量不足）；皮肤温度和肤色；毛细血管充盈延迟；黄疸（肝肾综合征）。

头眼耳鼻喉：口腔黏膜湿润，眼部湿润，颈静脉扁平（容量下降），静脉怒张（心力衰竭）。

胸部：湿啰音（心力衰竭）。

Heart: Irregular rhythm, murmurs, S3 (volume overload).

Abdomen: Hepatomegaly, abdominojugular reflux (heart failure); costovertebral angle tenderness; distended bladder, nephromegaly (obstruction).

Pelvic: Pelvic masses, cystocele, urethrocele.

Rectal: Prostate hypertrophy; absent sphincter reflex, decreased sensation (atonic bladder due to vertebral disk herniation).

Extremities: Peripheral edema (heart failure).

6. Labs

Sodium, potassium, BUN, creatinine, uric acid. Urine and serum osmolality, UA, urine creatinine. Ultrasound of bladder and kidneys.

7. Differential Diagnosis of Acute Renal Failure

Prerenal Insult:

Prerenal insult is the most common cause of acute renal failure, accounting for 70%. It is usually caused by reduced renal perfusion pressure secondary to extracellular fluid volume loss (diarrhea, diuresis, GI hemorrhage), or secondary to extracellular fluid sequestration (pancreatitis, sepsis), inadequate cardiac output, renal vasoconstriction (sepsis, liver disease), or inadequate fluid intake or replacement.

Intrarenal Insult:

(1) Insult to the renal parenchyma (tubular necrosis) causes 20% of acute renal failure.

(2) Prolonged hypoperfusion is the most common cause of tubular necrosis. Nephrotoxins (radiographic contrast, aminoglycosides) are the second most common cause of tubular necrosis.

(3) Pigmenturia induced renal injury can be caused by intravascular hemolysis or rhabdomyolysis.

(4) Acute glomerulonephritis or acute interstitial nephritis (usually from allergic reactions to beta-lactam antibiotics, sulfonamides, rifampin, NSAIDs, cimetidine, phenytoin, allopurinol, thiazides, furosemide, analgesics) are occasional causes of intrarenal kidney failure.

心脏：心律不齐，杂音，S3 奔马律（容量超负荷）。

腹部：肝肿大，腹颈静脉反流征（心力衰竭）；肋脊角压痛；膀胱扩张，肾肿大（梗阻）。

骨盆：盆腔肿块，膀胱膨出，尿道膨出。

直肠：前列腺肥大；括约肌反射消失，感觉下降（椎间盘突出致膀胱无力）。

四肢：外周水肿（心力衰竭）。

6. 实验室检查

钠，钾，尿素氮，肌酐，尿酸。尿液和血浆渗透压，尿常规，尿肌酐。膀胱和肾脏的超声检查。

7. 急性肾衰鉴别诊断

肾前性：

肾前性肾衰是急性肾衰最常见原因，占 70%。它常因细胞外液量丢失（腹泻，利尿，胃肠道出血）或细胞外液隔离（胰腺炎，败血症），心输出量不足，肾血管收缩（败血症，肝病）液体摄入或交换不足等所致的继发性肾灌注压降低所致。

肾性：

（1）20% 的急性肾衰竭是肾实质性（肾小管坏死）病变所致。

（2）长时间灌注不足是肾小管坏死的最常见原因。肾毒素药物（造影剂，氨基糖苷类）是肾小管坏死的第二大常见原因。

（3）色素尿所致肾损伤可由血管内溶血或横纹肌溶解引起。

（4）急性肾小球肾炎或急性间质性肾炎（通常来自对 β-内酰胺类抗生素，磺酰胺，利福平，非甾体抗炎药，西咪替丁，苯妥英钠，别嘌醇，噻嗪类，呋塞米，镇痛药的过敏反应）是肾衰竭的偶发原因。

Postrenal Insult:

(1) Postrenal damage results from obstruction of urine flow, and it is the least common cause of acute renal failure, accounting for 10%.

(2) Postrenal insult may be caused by prostate cancer, benign prostatic hypertrophy, renal calculi obstruction or amyloidosis, uric acid crystals, multiple myeloma, or acyclovir.

肾后性：

（1）肾后性肾衰是由尿流阻塞引起的，是急性肾衰竭的最少见原因，占 10%。

（2）可由前列腺癌，良性前列腺增生，肾结石阻塞或淀粉样变性，尿酸结晶，多发性骨髓瘤或阿昔洛韦引起。

十九、头晕&眩晕（Dizziness & Vertigo）

1. Chief Complaint

The patient is a 65-year-old female with hypertension who complains of dizziness for 1 hour.

2. History of the Present Illness

Sensation of spinning or movement of surroundings, light headedness, nausea, vomiting, tinnitus. Rate of onset of vertigo. Aggravation by change in position, turning head, changing from supine to standing, coughing. Hyperventilation, recent change in eyeglasses. Headache, hearing loss, head trauma, diplopia.

3. Past Medical History

Recent upper respiratory infection, paresthesia, syncope; hypertension, diabetes, history of stroke, transient ischemic attack, anemia, cardiovascular disease.

4. Medications Associated with Vertigo

Antihypertensives, aspirin, alcohol, sedatives, diuretics, phenytoin, gentamicin, furosemide.

5. Physical Examination

General Appearance: Effect of hyperventilation on symptoms. Effect of Valsalva maneuver on symptoms.

Vital Signs: Pulse, BP (supine and upright, postural hypotension), respiratory rate, temperature.

HEENT: Nystagmus, visual acuity, visual field deficits, papilledema; facial weakness. Tympanic membrane inflammation (otitis media), cerumen. Effect of head turning or of placing the patient recumbent with head extended over edge of bed; Rinne's test (air/bone conduction); Weber test (lateralization of sound).

十九、头晕＆眩晕

1. 主　诉

65 岁女性，高血压，患者头晕 1 小时。

2. 现病史

感觉周围环境旋转或运动，头晕，恶心，呕吐，耳鸣。眩晕的发生频率。因姿势变化，转头，仰卧变为站立，咳嗽而加重。换气过度，近期更换眼镜。头痛，听力下降，头部外伤，复视。

3. 既往史

近期上呼吸道感染，感觉异常，晕厥；高血压，糖尿病，中风，短暂性脑缺血发作，贫血，心血管疾病等病史。

4. 眩晕相关的药物

降压药，阿司匹林，酒精，镇静剂，利尿剂，苯妥英钠，庆大霉素，呋塞米。

5. 体格检查

一般情况：过度换气、Valsalva 动作对症状的影响。

生命体征：脉搏，血压（仰卧和直立，直立性低血压），呼吸频率，体温。

头眼耳鼻喉：眼震，视力，视野缺损，视乳头水肿；面部无力。鼓膜炎症（中耳炎），耵聍。转头或患者平躺，头部伸过床沿的影响；Rinne 试验（空气/骨传导）；Weber 试验（声音横向传导）。

Heart: Rhythm, murmurs.

Neuro: Cranial nerves 2-12, sensory deficits, ataxia, weakness. Romberg test, finger to nose test (coordination), tandem gait.

Rectal: Occult blood.

6. Labs

CBC, electrolytes, MRI scan.

7. Differential Diagnosis

Drugs Associated with Vertigo: Aminoglycosides, loop diuretics, aspirin, caffeine, alcohol, phenytoin, psychotropics (lithium, haloperidol), benzodiazepines.

Peripheral Causes of Vertigo: Acute labyrinthitis/neuronitis, benign positional vertigo, Meniere's disease (vertigo, tinnitus, deafness), otitis media, acoustic neuroma, cerebellopontine angle tumor, cholesteatoma (chronic middle ear effusion), impacted cerumen.

Central Causes of Vertigo: Vertebrobasilar insufficiency, brain stem or cerebellar infarctions, tumors, encephalitis, meningitis, brain stem or cerebellar contusion, Parkinson's disease, multiple sclerosis.

Other Disorders Associated with Vertigo: Motion sickness, presyncope, syndrome of multiple sensory deficits (peripheral neuropathies, visual impairment, orthopedic problems), new eyeglasses, orthostatic hypotension.

心脏：心律，杂音。

神经系统：颅神经 2-12，感觉缺陷，共济失调，无力。 Romberg 试验，指鼻试验（协调），踵趾步态。

直肠：隐血。

6. 实验室检查

血常规，电解质，MRI 扫描。

7. 鉴别诊断

眩晕有关的药物：氨基糖苷类，襻利尿剂，阿司匹林，咖啡因，酒精，苯妥英钠，精神药物（锂，氟哌啶醇），苯二氮卓类。

外周性眩晕：急性迷路炎/神经炎，良性位置性眩晕，美尼尔氏病（眩晕，耳鸣，耳聋），中耳炎，听神经瘤，小脑桥脑角肿瘤，胆脂瘤（慢性中耳积液），嵌顿性耵聍。

中枢性眩晕：椎基底动脉供血不足，脑干或小脑梗死，肿瘤，脑炎，脑膜炎，脑干或小脑挫伤，帕金森病，多发性硬化症。

其他疾病：晕动病，晕厥前期，多种感觉缺陷综合征（周围神经病变，视力障碍，骨科问题），新眼镜，直立性低血压。

二十、意识模糊、谵妄&昏迷（Confusion, Delirium & Coma）

1. Chief Complaint

The patient is a 70-year-old male with coronary heart disease who presents with confusion for 6 hours.

2. History of the Present Illness

Level of consciousness, obtundation (awake but not alert), stupor (unconscious but arousable with vigorous pain or verbal stimulation), coma (cannot be awakened). Confusion, hallucination; poor concentration, agitation. Activity and symptoms prior to onset. Fever, headache, epilepsy (post-ictal state).

3. Past Medical History

Trauma, suicide attempts or depression, dementia, stroke, transient ischemic attacks, hypertension; renal, liver or cardiac disease.

4. Medications

Insulin, oral hypoglycemics, narcotics, alcohol, drugs, antipsychotics, anticholinergics, anticoagulant.

5. Physical Examination

General Appearance: Signs of dehydration, septic appearance.

Vital Signs: BP (hypertensive encephalopathy), pulse, temperature (fever), respiratory rate.

HEENT: Skull palpation for tenderness, lacerations. Pupil size and reactivity; extraocular movements. Papilledema, hemorrhages, flame lesions; facial asymmetry, ptosis, weakness. Battle's sign (ecchymosis over mastoid process), raccoon sign (periorbital ecchymosis, skull fracture), hemotympanum (basal skull fracture). Tongue or cheek lacerations (post-ictal state). Atrophic tongue (vitamin B_{12} deficiency).

Neck: Neck rigidity, carotid bruits.

二十、意识模糊，谵妄和昏迷

1. 主 诉

70 岁男性，冠心病患者，意识模糊 6 小时。

2. 现病史

意识水平，迟钝（清醒但不警觉），昏睡（意识不清但在强烈刺激下可觉醒），昏迷（无法觉醒）。意识模糊，幻觉；注意力不集中，情绪激动。发病前的活动和症状。发热，头痛，癫痫（发作后状态）。

3. 既往史

创伤，自杀未遂或抑郁，痴呆，中风，短暂性脑缺血发作，高血压；肾脏，肝脏或心脏疾病。

4. 药物史

胰岛素，口服降糖药，麻醉剂，酒精，药物，抗精神病药，抗胆碱药，抗凝药。

5. 体格检查

一般情况：脱水迹象，败血症外观。

生命体征：血压（高血压脑病），脉搏，体温（发热），呼吸频率。

头眼耳鼻喉：颅骨触痛，裂伤。瞳孔大小和对光反射；眼外肌运动。视乳头水肿，出血，火焰样病变；面部不对称，上睑下垂，无力。Battle 征（乳突瘀斑），熊猫征（眶周瘀斑，颅骨骨折），鼓室出血（颅底骨折）。舌或颊裂伤（癫痫发作后状态）。舌头萎缩（维生素 B_{12} 缺乏症）。

颈部：颈部僵硬，颈动脉杂音。

Chest: Breathing pattern (Cheyne-Stokes hyperventilation); crackles, wheezes.

Heart: Rhythm, murmurs.

Abdomen: Hepatomegaly, splenomegaly, masses, ascites, tenderness, distention, dilated superficial veins (liver failure).

Extremities: Needle track marks (drug overdose), tattoos.

Skin: Cyanosis, jaundice, spider angiomata, palmarerythema (hepatic encephalopathy); capillary refill, petechia, splinter hemorrhages. Injection site fat atrophy (diabetes).

Neuro: Concentration (subtraction of serial 7s, delirium), strength, cranial nerves 2-12, mini-mental status exam; orientation to person, place, time, recent events; Babinski's sign, primitive reflexes (snout, suck, glabella, palmomental grasp). Tremor (Parkinson's disease, delirium tremens), incoherent speech, lethargy, somnolence.

Glasgow Coma Scale

(1) Best Verbal Response:

None: 1; incomprehensible sounds or cries: 2; appropriate words or vocal sounds: 3; confused speech or words: 4; oriented speech: 5.

(2) Best Eye Opening Response:

No eye opening: 1; eyes open to pain: 2; eyes open to speech: 3; eyes open spontaneously: 4.

(3) Best Motor Response:

None: 1; abnormal extension to pain: 2; abnormal flexion to pain: 3; withdraws to pain: 4; localizes to pain: 5; obeys commands: 6.

Total Score: 3-15.

6. Labs

Glucose, electrolytes, calcium, BUN, creatinine, ABG. CT/MRI, ammonia, alcohol, liver function tests, urine toxicology screen, B-12, folate levels. LP if no signs of elevated intracranial pressure and suspicion of meningitis.

胸部：呼吸方式（Cheyne-Stokes 过度换气）；湿啰音，喘息声。

心脏：心律，杂音。

腹部：肝肿大，脾肿大，肿块，腹水，压痛，扩张，浅表静脉扩张（肝衰竭）。

肢体：针刺痕迹（药物过量），纹身。

皮肤：发绀，黄疸，蜘蛛痣，肝掌（肝性脑病）；毛细血管充盈，瘀斑，裂片样出血。注射部位脂肪萎缩（糖尿病）。

神经系统：注意力（连续减 7，谵妄），力量，颅神经 2-12，微精神状态检查；人，地方，时间定向力，最近事件；Babinski 的体征，原始反射（鼻部，吮吸，眉间，掌颏反射）。震颤（帕金森病，谵妄），言语不连贯，昏睡，嗜睡。

格拉斯哥昏迷量表

（1）言语反应：

无反应：1 分；难理解的声音或哭声：2 分；可说单词或声音：3 分；答非所问：4 分；言语条理清晰：5 分。

（2）睁眼反应：

无睁眼：1 分；疼痛睁眼：2 分；呼唤睁眼：3 分；自然睁眼：4 分。

（3）肢体反应：

无反应：1 分；遇疼痛肢体伸直：2 分；遇疼痛肢体屈曲：3 分；遇疼痛肢体缩回：4 分；遇疼痛可定位：5 分；遵守动作命令：6 分。

总分：3 ~ 15 分。

6．实验室检查

血糖，电解质，钙，尿素氮，肌酐，动脉血气分析。CT/MRI，血氨，酒精，肝功能检查，尿毒物学筛查，维生素 B_{12}，叶酸水平。腰穿：若怀疑脑膜炎且无颅内压升高。

7. Differential Diagnosis of Delirium

Electrolyte imbalance, hyperglycemia, hypoglycemia (insulin overdose), alcohol or drug withdraw or intoxication, hypoxia, meningitis, encephalitis, systemic infection, stroke, intracranial hemorrhage, postictal state, exacerbation of dementia; narcotic or anticholinergic overdose; steroid withdrawal, hepatic encephalopathy; psychotic states, dehydration, hypertensive encephalopathy, head trauma, subdural hematoma, uremia, vitamin B_{12} or folate deficiency, hypothyroidism, ketoacidosis, factitious coma.

7. 谵妄鉴别诊断

电解质紊乱，高血糖症，低血糖症（胰岛素过量），戒酒或中毒，缺氧，脑膜炎，脑炎，全身感染，中风，颅内出血，癫痫发作后状态，痴呆加剧；麻醉或抗胆碱药过量；类固醇停药，肝性脑病；精神病状态，脱水，高血压脑病，头部外伤，硬脑膜下血肿，尿毒症，维生素 B_{12} 或叶酸缺乏，甲状腺功能低下，酮症酸中毒，人为性昏迷。

参考文献（Reference）

[1] FAREH S. English for medicine & health sciences[M]. Amsterdam: Elsevier, 2017.

[2] BALL J W, DAINS J E, FLYNN J A, et al. Seidel's guide to physical examination — an interprofessional approach[M]. 9th Ed. Amsterdam: Elsevier Inc, 2019.

[3] GLENDINNING E H, HOLMSTRÖM B A S. English in medicine[M]. 3rd Ed. Cambridge: Cambridge University Press, 2005.

[4] EHRLICH A, SCHRÖDER C L, EHRLICH L, et al. Terminology for health professions[M]. 8th Ed. Stamford: CENGAGE Learning, 2016.

[5] ROTER D L, HALL J A. Doctors talking with patients patients talking with doctors improving communication in medical visits[M]. 2nd Ed. SanFrancisco: Praeger, 2006.

[6] KUMAR N, LAW A. Teaching rounds a visual aid to teaching internal medicine PEARLS on the WARDS[M]. New York: McGraw-Hill Education, 2016.

[7] JEVON P, ODOGWU S. Medical student survival skills history taking and communication skills[M]. New Jersey: Wiley Blackwell, 2020.

[8] MARSHALL S, RUEDY J. On call principles and protocols[M]. 6th Ed. Amsterdam: Elsevier, 2016.

附录（Appendix）

常用缩写

ac = ante cibum (before meals)

ABG = arterial blood gas

AFB = acid-fast bacillus

ALT = alanine aminotransferase

am = morning

amp = ampule

ANA = antinuclear antibody

ante = before

AP = anteroposterior

ARDS = adult respiratory distress syndrome

AST = aspartate aminotransferase

bid = bis in die (twice a day)

B-12 = vitamin B_{12} (cyanocobalamin)

BMP = basic metabolic panel

BP = blood pressure

bpm = breaths per minute, beats per minute

BUN = blood urea nitrogen

c/o = complaint of

c = cum (with)

C and S = culture and sensitivity

C = centigrade

Ca = calcium

cap = capsule

CBC = complete blood count

cc = cubic centimeter

CCU = coronary care unit

cm = centimeter

CNS = central nervous system

CO_2 = carbon dioxide

COPD = chronic obstructive pulmonary disease

CK-MB = myocardial-specific CPK isoenzyme

CPR = cardiopulmonary resuscitation

CT = computerized tomography

CVP = central venous pressure

CXR = Chest X-ray

d/c = discharge; discontinue

DIC = disseminated intravascular coagulation

diff = differential count

DKA = diabetic ketoacidosis

dL = deciliter

DTs = delirium tremens

ECG = electrocardiogram

ER = emergency room

ERCP = endoscopic retrograde cholangiopancreatography

ESR = erythrocyte sedimentation rate

ET = endotracheal tube

FEV1 = forced expiratory volume (in one second)

FiO_2 = fractional inspired oxygen

g = gram(s)

GFR = glomerular filtration rate

GI = gastrointestinal

gm = gram

gt = drop

gtt = drops

h = hour

H_2O = water

HBsAG = hepatitis B surface antigen

HCO_3^- = bicarbonate

Hct = hematocrit

HDL = high-density lipoprotein

Hg = mercury

Hgb = hemoglobin concentration

HIV = human immunodeficiency virus

hr = hour

IM = intramuscular

I and O = intake and output

I&D = incision&drainage

IU = international units

ICU = intensive care unit

IgM = immunoglobulin M

IMV = intermittent mandatory ventilation

INR = International normalized ratio

IV = intravenous or intravenously

K^+ = potassium

kcal = kilocalorie

KCL = potassium chloride

KH_2PO_4 = potassium phosphate

KUB = kidneys, ureters, bowels (X-ray of abdomen)

L = liter

LDH = lactate dehydrogenase

LDL = low-density lipoprotein

liq = liquid

LLQ = left lower quadrant

LP = lumbar puncture, low potency

LR = lactated Ringer's (solution)

MBC = minimal bacterial concentration

mcg = microgram

mEq = milliequivalent

mg = milligram

Mg = magnesium

$MgSO_4$ = Magnesium Sulfate

MI = myocardial infarction

MIC = minimum inhibitory concentration

mL = milliliter

Mm = millimeter

MRI = magnetic resonance imaging

Na = sodium

$NaHCO_3$ = sodium bicarbonate

Neuro = neurologic

NG = nasogastric

NKA = no known allergies

NS = normal saline solution (0.9%)

NSAID = nonsteroidal anti-inflammatory drug

O_2 = oxygen

Osm = osmolality

OT = occupational therapy

OTC = over the counter

P = post, after

pc = post cibum (after meals)

PA = posteroanterior; pulmonary artery

PaO_2 = arterial oxygen pressure

pAO_2 = partial pressure of oxygen in alveolar gas

PB = phenobarbital

pCO_2 = partial pressure of carbon dioxide

PEEP = positive end-expiratory pressure

pH = hydrogen ion concentration (H^+)

pm = afternoon

PMI = the point of maximal impulse

PO = orally, per os

pO_2 = partial pressure of oxygen

PR = per rectum

prn = pro re nata (as needed)

PT = physical therapy; prothrombin time

PTCA = percutaneous transluminal coronary angioplasty

PTT = partial thromboplastin time

PVC = premature ventricular contraction

q = quaque (every)

q6h = every 6 hours

q2h = every 2 hours

qid = quarter in die (four times a day)

qAM = every morning

qd = quaque die (every day)

qh = every hour

qhs = every night before bedtime

qid = 4 times a day

qOD = every other day

qs = quantity sufficient

R/O = rule out

RA = rheumatoid arthritis;

Resp = respiratory rate

RL = Ringer's lactated solution (also LR)

ROM = range of motion

sat = saturated

SBP = systolic blood pressure

SC = subcutaneously

SL = sublingually under tongue

SLE = systemic lupus erythematosus

sob = shortness of breath

sol = solution

susp = suspension

tid = ter in die (three times a day)

T4 = Thyroxine level (T4)

tab = tablet

TB = tuberculosis

Temp = temperature

TIA = transient ischemic attack

tid = three times a day

TSH = thyroid-stimulating hormone

U = units

URI = upper respiratory infection

UTI = urinary tract infection